The Joys and Tears of a Doctor

10-31-95

To Denise
Who has found joy in
being a neighbor to my
patient Sharon

Timothy h Curran MD

The Joys and Tears of a Doctor

How Irish Humor, Dedicated Care
and Strong Faith Help to
Solve Patients' Problems

by

Timothy L. Curran, M.D.

Woodstock Books
Plainville, CT

Library of Congress Catalog Card Number 98-61364

ISBN 0-9640096-5-X

Printed in Canada
First Printing 1998

Published by
Woodstock Books
Plainville, CT

Contents

To my wife, Mary,who walked many miles with me during our courtship days. She was forced to walk alone during my two years of overseas duty. She followed my steps to help establish our home far from her family and friends when we decided to plant our roots in Hartford. Her love and true faith smoothed out the rough and sometimes rocky road that slowed but did not stop our progress to a happy, satisfying life. She established relationships with professional and nonprofessional friends that became steadfast and strong through all the years.

To my children, Timothy, John, and Elizabeth, who found the same joy in orienting themselves to the medical care of people that was first experienced by their mother in her nursing career and shared by all of us as I progressed through my years of practice. No father could ask for more love than they bestowed on me despite my forced absence on many special family occasions.

Acknowledgements

My thanks are extended to many people who gave me help and encouragement during the writing of this book. Two individuals to whom I'm especially indebted are my sisters, Mary McGunnigle and Rita Sands. They jogged my memory in many ways and supplied the names and dates relating to various incidents that developed during our early family life.

To Boston College goes my special gratitude for providing me with the groundwork of an education and principles which carried me successfully through my medical training and practice.

To Boston University Medical School for accepting me as a student and giving me the fundamentals which inspired me to become a member of the most prestigious societies of my medical specialty.

I feel indebted to Lowell Stone for initiating a course of instruction in creative writing which I was fortunate enough to attend. His guidance and stimulation inspired a good number of men and women to reveal a talent that otherwise would have remained dormant. Robert Spencer, a retired clergyman and a member of the class, took over the leadership of the group following the tragic death of Lowell Stone. "Spence" continued to carry on the monthly sessions for interested writers in the same grand tradition as our respected teacher.

I shall never forget Medical Economics, a national magazine distributed to physicians, for publishing a number of my articles. The editor's acceptance of my anecdotal experiences stimulated me to go further and finally to write a book describing the interesting and exciting events of a physician's life.

And to Dr. Edward Zebrowski goes a special thanks. His unwavering confidence in my ability to complete this book was exactly what I needed to keep working on the manuscript.

I extend my deepest appreciation to all the above and to many others who have influenced my writing in so many different ways.

Timothy L. Curran, M.D.
Avon, Connecticut

1
PROLOGUE

My Family

The history of our country is filled with the hardships endured by those who sought a better life than they had been experiencing in their homeland. The small band of Puritans who settled in Massachusetts in 1620 chafed under the restrictions of the Church of England and found their religious freedom in the New World.

Other groups followed from England, Scotland, and Ireland as well as the rest of the European continent, seeking an escape from a life that offered little hope for their future. The emigration from Ireland began to accelerate in the early 1800s and became a mass exodus in the 1840s when the potato famine caused starvation with death to millions.

In 1891 at the age of 13, my mother, Mary Naughton, left Ireland for America with her cousin, Kate Naughton, who was the same age. Unlike most young Irish who emigrated to this country, these intrepid young ladies did not stop in Boston or New York but proceeded directly to California. This was all arranged by an uncle, Pat King, who paid for all their travel arrangements.

It was not unusual in the late 19th century and early 1900s for many young Irish lads to leave their homestead and seek their fortune in America. Once their roots were set in this new country they sponsored other family members to join them. My wife's father, Martin Earley, followed this same routine after he emigrated to Boston at the turn of the century. The Earley family would frequently have several relatives living in their crowded household. Once the newcomers became established in jobs, often obtained with the help of Martin Earley, they found their own living quarters. For several years the Earley home had a succession of Irish cousins who stayed on until work was obtained and they settled into their own lodging.

Pat King did not stop off in New York or Boston where most young Irish decided to reside. He apparently set out immediately for California where he soon became successful in real estate and encouraged other members of the family to follow his path of success.

Uncle Pat enrolled Mary Naughton and Kate at the Dominican Academy where they completed the equivalent of a high school education. Live-in employment at the Santa Barbara home of Robert Dollar, who owned the Dollar Steamship Line, was also arranged for by Pat King. The house duties included cleaning and laundry work with adequate time for her studies. At the age of 18, Mary Naughton decided to return to Ireland but her cousin Kate stayed on, eventually married and established her home in Palo Alto. My mother frequently mentioned how kind the Dollar family had been to her. However, homesickness apparently overcame her and she left California and became reunited with her family and friends in Spiddal.

In 1897 my father, whose name was Timothy, left his hometown of Spiddal, settled in Boston and shortly afterwards became a citizen. It was a pattern followed by many Irish as it helped to build up a solid block of voters that eventually toppled the Brahmins from power. It was 2 years later that my mother also departed from her home in Spiddal and married my father at St Augustine's Church in South Boston.

My father being the oldest son of a family that numbered 12 children, was notified that the family farm was bequeathed to him at the death of his father in 1900. My father and mother returned to Spiddal where they took over the active cultivation of the farm. The decision to spend life on the farm was soon determined to be unwise and within a year my father gave up ownership of the acreage to the next brother in line. A short time later Timothy and Mary Curran returned to America and once again my father renewed his employment with the City of Boston Public Works Department.

RISING FROM POVERTY

A Family Miracle

"Three-year-old John Curran was cured of paralysis following visits to St. Leonard's Church in the north end of Boston."

This yellowed news item from the Boston Post was shown to the family some years afterwards and we all agreed that a miracle had occurred.

My mother related what had happened.

"John awakened one morning and I noticed he was dragging his right leg. When no improvement occurred after several days I decided to bring him to the Boston City hospital."

This huge municipal hospital had become recognized for the treatment of many diseases and was a mecca for the indigent as well as the middle class of Greater Boston. The diagnosis of infantile paralysis (later identified as poliomyelitis) was established and for many weeks there were regular family visits to the hospital. However, despite the recommended treatment of massage and warm soaks no improvement was noted over a period of six months.

My mother was a very religious woman and she finally determined that help from a higher authority was needed.

"I had prayed he would get better, but finally I brought him to St. Leonard's Church, also know as the 'Miracle Church.' For two months there was no change despite weekly visits to the basilica. One morning I noticed that he walked without any dragging of his leg."

When the rest of the family was shown the newspaper clipping we were duly impressed, but we also asked what the doctors thought.

"I took him back to the City Hospital and they agreed he had no paralysis and pronounced him cured. They had no answer as to why he showed a perfectly normal-functioning right leg since their last examination several months earlier."

It was after this last hospital visit that my mother reported the miracle to the church authorities. The newspaper article followed. Following my birth several years later, I was given the middle name of Leonard in honor of the miraculous saint.

Medicine is filled with stories of unexplained recoveries from illnesses that seem to defy the best efforts of the physician to effect a cure. The unbelievers will discount the miraculous events. The faithful will credit their improvement or recovery to God's help.

The danger is the failure, at times, to seek medical attention when the disease process might be fatal unless proper attention is given to the victim along with the recourse to the Lord. This is a problem that any individual faces when his faith takes precedence over logic such as may occur in Christian Science or when dealing with faith healers.

My mother and the doctors saw no improvement in my brother John's condition during his months of treatment. Her decision to seek help from a higher authority was certainly justified and his response to divine intervention is difficult to question.

Death Visits our Young Family

"Hail Mary full of grace, the Lord is with thee."

As the priest led the prayers for my mother at Dolan's Funeral Home, it was a repetition of the supplication that was delivered in the same room 25 years earlier, when my father died. As I gazed down at my mother's face, there was a serenity that sometimes only death can bring. I felt a lump in my throat and tears in my eyes as I recalled the events that had led to the loss of the family breadwinner in December 1920.

"Call the City Hospital. It is urgent."

The telephone message received at McDermott's Variety Store across the street brought an immediate response from my mother. She returned in a few minutes and gathered my sisters and brothers around her and solemnly gave us the shocking news.

"Daddy is dead and I must go to the hospital tonight," she said.

It was now 9 PM, but before leaving she made sure that we were all tucked into bed. She gave instructions to my eleven-year-old brother, John, to watch over us until she returned. The trip to the hospital was an hour's journey by street car. On this sub-zero December night my mother reinforced her winter coat with a heavy muffler to ward off the blustery winds we heard howling outside our windows as we lay wide-awake in our beds in the darkness of the night.

When my mother returned several hours later, we were still awake, even my two-year-old sister, Rita, but the news was good.

"Daddy has not died, but he is very sick," my mother said quietly.

With this news we all kneeled down and said a prayer of thanksgiving and peacefully went to sleep. The following evening, sometime after 10 PM, the same message was received from the neighborhood store. Another sorrowful trip to the hospital for my mother ended with the news that my father had indeed died and the reality of being a widow with five children from the age of two to eleven now had to be faced.

Influenza, the cause of death for many millions throughout the world in previous epidemics, had recurred in 1920 after being relatively dormant for several years. My father became one of many thousands who died in Boston, New York, and other metropolitan areas along the East Coast that same year. This highly contagious viral infection invaded the lungs, bringing on an overwhelming pneumonia. The thick secretions that blocked the bronchial tubes prevented the flow of any air and suffocation ensued.

There were no antibiotics, no vaccines, and no chest pumps to help the victims to breathe. The influenza virus was no respecter of people since it affected the rich and the poor, the strong and the weak, the young and the old.

Living in the poorer section of Dorchester, a suburb of Boston, there was always a constant struggle "to keep a roof over our heads and three meals on the table." The meager wages earned by my father driving a city dump truck provided bare sustenance and nothing else. The death of the breadwinner left the family with no pension fund, social security, nor other financial sources to ease the burden of a widow with children. With no savings, the only recourse for my mother was city welfare, known as the Overseers of the Poor. This support became a gateway to freedom from hunger and a bridge to a life in the future that we were all privileged to enjoy. I have been forever grateful for this help. During my later productive years, one of my priorities was a tithing of my income for a wide spectrum of charities.

Despite the equivalent of a high school education, my mother could only find employment performing menial household tasks. She made herself available for work in the homes of those who lived in the upper class community of Milton several miles distant. When my father died, I was seven-years-old and my sisters were two and four. My brother Francis was nine and John was eleven. During those first few years we were fortunate in having good neighbors.

They supervised my sisters while the boys attended school and my mother was given the opportunity of working a few extra hours, thus lessening her dependence on the welfare roles.

The story of survival for most deprived families is filled with sacrifices and hard work.

The individuals who experience such tragedy will agree their success in later life can be traced to facing reality. Only by hard work can they find their way out of the pit's bottom. In our family we had John, my older brother, who became the father surrogate of the family at the age of eleven. It was John who would find jobs as a newsboy, then delivery boy for the local grocery story, and later as a drugstore clerk. All of these positions were inherited by me as I moved up his ladder of success.

It was one year after my father's death that my mother's sister, Eliza Clancy, lost her 21-year-old son, Joseph, to uncontrollable diabetes. Aunt Lizzie lived in Ireland and had become a widow several years earlier. The discovery of insulin by Frederick Grant Banting of Canada was a year too late to save the life of her only child.

My mother received many entreaties from her sister who wrote at first asking, then later demanding that one of the boys, preferably John or Francis, be sent to Ireland to help on the farm.

After several years of such correspondence, my mother agreed to send Francis, who was eleven-years-old at that time. The decision must have been a difficult and traumatic one for my mother, but to my knowledge she never discussed it with us and we never inquired. At that time our ages were four to thirteen, which didn't qualify us to help in giving any opinions. The motivating factor, undoubtedly, was the reality of feeding one child who was needed more desperately by an aunt who could provide for him more adequately.

The Relatives

"Uncle Tom is sick and you can't use the bathroom."

When my aunt said this to me I went home as she suggested. It was sometime later, after telling my mother what had happened, that I also mentioned the strong odor coming from the closed bathroom door. My mother made no comment, but the mystery was solved when the incident was related to my ten-year-old, always knowledgeable, brother John and he explained what was taking place.

"Uncle Tom makes home brew in the bath tub," John said.

Making home brew was a common practice as I learned after my brother's explanation. On subsequent visits to the Kelly home I was sometimes aware of the same odor, but I never asked to use the bathroom unless the door was open.

We did have other relatives, the Costellos, who lived several streets away. Close by their house was a large open field where the neighborhood youngsters played ball. I would often see Uncle Mike coming home from work and noticed he seemed to walk with a staggering gait. In my childhood ignorance I thought my uncle had a leg or hip problem. Later I happened to mention this observation to John, who quickly told me the reason for Uncle Mike's problem.

"Uncle Mike stops by the local tavern before he gets to his house. He often stays longer than he should and he can't walk very straight after he leaves the tavern."

Uncle Mike and Uncle Tom married my father's sisters and despite my mother's attempts to maintain a friendly relationship, we rarely shared any family social events. The lack of hospitality became more evident after my father died.

Whenever my mother conversed with friends or neighbors, she always expressed herself clearly and in a reasonably articulate manner. This undoubtedly created jealousy and resentment with her sisters-in-law who certainly did not have the gift of speech or knowledge possessed by my mother. During our years at the local grade schools, John and I as well as my sisters, always attained top grades which continued through high school and allowed us to be accepted into college. My mother was proud of our accomplishments, but there was no doubt that our scholastic achievements must have caused considerable annoyance to the relatives who found their children lagging behind.

Losing my First Job

One of my duties at O'Keefe's Grocery Store after school and Saturdays was the delivery of orders to customers in the neighborhood. This became my job at the age of eight after John found work at Archer's Drug Store.

It was two years later that disaster struck after visiting the O'Meara home about one mile from the store. The unpredictable weather of March had been ushered in that day by a real nor'easter with heavy snow and biting winds. The piled-up groceries were covered with the snow that was coming down rapidly and the drifts were already deep on the streets and sidewalks as I trudged towards my forthcoming misfortune. These were the days when the only roads being plowed were those used by the streetcars. Even before the famous quotation, years later attributed to Mayor James Curley, it was accepted that "God gave us the snow. Let God take it away."

It took three trips to the top floor of the three-decker house to reach and unload the grocery order from the sled. Mrs. O'Meara, a huge woman with bare legs distended by fat and varicosities, sat back in her rocker watching me intently as I set the bags on the kitchen table.

Her son, Martin, also surveyed what was taking place and like his mother, he too was grossly overweight. He also had a fat mouth which caused me to have several encounters with him at school.

"Mama, look at the groceries," he said. "They're all wet."

I was annoyed by Martin's comments about the wet bags since there was no way that the groceries could be protected from the snow-lined streets and sidewalks or the continuing falling flakes.

Mrs. O'Meara now added to my torment by shouting, "I'll report you to the manager."

The next day I took out my anger on Martin as he walked ahead of me after class. Joined by eager friends who also disliked him, Martin became the object of snow balls that continually caught up with him as he ran and stumbled to his home. It was several days later that the grocery manager advised me that Mrs. O'Meara's complaints forced him to take action and I lost my position as delivery boy. It was an early lesson in learning the hard way that restraint must be exercised if you expect to get ahead successfully in life.

Greasing Engines on the Railroad

John Reen was a general foreman of the New Haven Railroad's engine roundhouse located on Dover Street in Boston. As a cousin of my mother's, he recognized the family financial plight and when my brother John turned fourteen, he found summer work for him as a laborer. Later, when I reached sixteen, he came to our rescue again and arranged my employment as a grease monkey and other sundry jobs around the engine roundhouse.

The work itself was rather dirty and laborious, but I enjoyed the camaraderie of those to whom I was assigned each day. I had some difficulty with only one mechanic, Whitey, who would frequently complain along with some curses about my assistance. Finally, I became really annoyed when he dropped a large wrench while he was working on a locomotive. With a string of stinging epithets, he yelled down to where I was doing some greasing chores. "Hey, you little jerk," he yelled out, "bring up that wrench I just dropped and snap to it."

He added a few expletives to his request.

My reply was instantaneous, but not appropriate.

"Pick it up yourself," I yelled back.

This infuriated Whitey. He spat down on me and it caught me squarely in the eye. I retrieved the tool which weighed three or four pounds and made another mistake. I hurled it with all my might at his head but fortunately missed. Whitey weighed well over 200 pounds. He started to come down towards me from the engine cab. I immediately grabbed a pointed shovel that was close by and prepared to defend myself. One of the boss foremen came along to see what the ruckus was all about. He told Whitey to get back to work. I never had any further trouble with Whitey. Later I learned that his animosity stemmed from his failure to get a friend the job that was given to me.

During those depression years I was fortunate to have my evening and weekend work at the drugstore along with the grease-monkey summer employment at the railroad during the day.

Subsequently, the WPA supplied me with construction jobs during my college and early medical school periods. The first year in construction was strictly 'pick and shovel.'

The following year I ran for delegate to the pre-primary Democratic Convention. There were twenty-four individuals running for three openings and I came in fourth. All was not lost since that summer I was given the job of timekeeper for a WPA project that was involved with building sidewalks leading to the Suffolk Downs Race Track. I'm not sure if anybody ever walked to the track, but the sidewalk was there for anybody who had the inclination.

Drugstore Clerking

My job at the drugstore began shortly after being dismissed from O'Keefe's as a delivery boy. It was year-round work that started at 7:30 in the morning when I opened up the store, washed the floor, filled the syrup and soda tanks at the fountain and left for school for my classes. In the evenings I usually started at 6:00 PM, finishing at the closing hour of 10:30. Saturday and Sundays my workday started at 8 AM and finished at 6 PM. When I was able to find full-time work in the summer, my drugstore clerking was restricted to evenings and Sundays.

A customer at the drugstore overheard me as I related my daytime summer activities to a friend. She berated me for having two positions while her husband was completely unemployed. I told her that I was ready to give up both jobs if someone would pay my tuition. I don't think that my explanation satisfied her.

In addition to working at the soda fountain and waiting on the customers for their sundry needs, I would grind up the materials which the pharmacist carefully placed in capsules to be dispensed according to the doctor's direction. Occasionally the prescriptions were delivered to the patients' homes by me, but most customers waited at the store until the medication was ready.

Lydia Pinkham's Compound was a popular item which was dispensed without a prescription. It was widely advertised as a tonic and cure for almost any female disorder and flourished for over half a century. In 1920 the Volstead Act became effective after being passed by Congress and became known as Prohibition. The alcoholic content of the Pinkham concoction was far beyond the alcoholic content of near beer, the sale of which was allowed by the Prohibition Law. Lydia's female tonic became the stimulating beverage of the laboring class. At the same time a group of Louisiana politicians formed a company that sold a tonic called Hadacol which had a higher alcoholic content than the Pinkham mixture. Hadacol became one of the drugstore's best-selling products, especially on Saturday, the workingman's payday. The Prohibitionists became aware of the subterfuge being used to bypass the

Volstead Act and Congress passed a law restricting the amount of alcohol allowed in so-called medicinal tonics.

The 18th Amendment, which prohibited the sale of alcoholic beverages, was repealed in 1933. By that time the reduced alcoholic contents of the medical tonics had long since lost their popularity.

During the period of alcoholic deprivation the upper class always had access to imported whiskeys through their personal bootleggers. The workingman was also able to find a bootlegger who supplied him with an intoxicating beverage. One of my bootlegger customers was a man named Dutch who was just over five-feet-tall with a cigarette always hanging from the corner of his mouth and his hat brim pulled down over one side of his face. I made a near-fatal mistake when Dutch came in one day and asked for a quart of glycerine which was located on a lower shelf next to the castor oil. I wrapped up the castor oil by mistake and the next day I was told by Dutch a gallon of grain alcohol had been ruined by my error. Fortunately, he only cussed me out and failed to take any physical action against me.

2
MEDICAL SCHOOL

Medical School Rejection and Acceptance

Worth Hale, the Dean of admissions at Harvard Medical School looked at me with obvious scorn and contempt.

"Your problem is that you went to the wrong school in the first place," he said sneeringly.

Those words should have immediately prompted me to walk out of the interview. Instead, I decided to stand my ground. I hoped to change his mind and attitude.

But Dr. Hale wasn't finished with his diatribe.

"Furthermore," he continued, "graduates of Boston College do not perform very well at Harvard Medical school."

Despite the realization that I was facing a bigot of the first magnitude, a rigid individual intolerantly devoted to his prejudices, I was not about to be put off in my quest for admission into medical school.

In an attempt to refute his statement, I replied, "I am acquainted with several of the recent graduates of Boston College who had been accepted to Harvard and know for a fact that they are doing excellent work."

It was common knowledge that Harvard had a quota of two students each year to be accepted from Boston College and Holy Cross, the two Jesuit colleges in Massachusetts. Usually, the top two premed students at Boston College were recommended each year by the head of the science department. To my knowledge no other students were accepted.

I had received my Bachelor's Degree from B.C. and that included some of the basic requirements for medical school. As is still true in most premed studies, the courses were heavily weighted in sciences. The latter included many hours of laboratory sessions which not only lengthened the day, but also increased the tuition costs. I could afford neither the extra expense nor the lengthened day which would have precluded my work at the drugstore.

My postgraduate year at Harvard University enabled me to fulfill the premedical requirements. It did not open doors to Harvard Medical School, however. The interview with Worth Hale left me somewhat crestfallen and of course, angry at his responses.

It was only a few days after my disastrous meeting with Hale that Dr. Roswell Ham dropped into the drugstore where I worked every weekend for the previous two years. My job as a clerk had begun many years earlier in the main store, but the weekend clerking at this satellite store, a mile distant, proved to be a godsend.

Dr. Ham had become a good friend and confidant during those few years that we became acquainted. Whenever he visited the store, he would spend a few moments to chat in some general small talk, but he was especially interested in my desire to become a doctor.

This tall, gray-haired old gentleman in his late 60s lived in an apartment close to the store. From our earlier conversations I knew that his office was located in the Back Bay area. This was an exclusive section of Boston and the favored location for the top medical specialists. During our many friendly chats I learned that his practice was restricted to gynecology.

My aspirations for a career in medicine were limited to finding acceptance to a medical school in Boston. Any institution in some other state would require finding a job that could also pay my tuition and supply enough return for living quarters and three meals a day. That was possible with my drugstore clerkship, but not likely to be found in some other state.

The only acceptable medical schools in Boston were Harvard, Tufts, and Boston University. There was one Grade C school, Middlesex, located in a deteriorating section of Boston. Its graduates had a 75-80% failure rate on the medical licensing exams and their training was totally inadequate. It was the end of the line for some who desired to become doctors but whose premedical training was markedly insufficient.

If I failed to gain admission to a Grade A medical school in Boston, my hopes for reaching my goal as a physician rested in either Tufts or BU. Clerking at the drugstore and living at home was my only financial salvation.

During one of my little chats with Dr. Ham he was most cordial when he asked me one day, "Are you still pursuing admission to medical school?"

Mentioning nothing about my miserable encounter with Dr. Hale, I told him that I was in the process of sending out my applications. It was then that he really raised my hopes and expectations.

"As a member of the teaching staff at BU, I am asked to review the applications of candidates for admission to the Medical School. When you fill out your application I will be happy to add a letter of recommendation."

Dr. Ham's supportive words were the answer to my prayers and I wasted no time in following his suggestion. Within two weeks a letter arrived from Boston University.

"We are pleased to inform you of your acceptance into Boston University Medical School."

I didn't need to read any further. That was all I wanted to know. I had made it and owed it all to Dr. Ham.

Why did Dr. Ham, with whom I had only what seemed a casual acquaintance, take such a fatherly interest in my desire to reach my objective in medicine? Perhaps there was something in me that attracted his attention and convinced him that I would make a good doctor. To him I have been forever grateful.

Some years after graduation another medical school classmate, Ken McClane, recounted his experience with Dr. Hale. Ken had an excellent record in college and was recommended by medical friends of his father who was a professor at Columbia University. Ken McClane later practiced medicine for many years in New York City and was the recipient of many outstanding awards for his service to the community.

His interview at Harvard ended abruptly when Worth Hale reviewed McClane's record and then made this pronouncement:

"Mr. McClane, you have done very well in college and we will admit you to Harvard, but only on one condition. You must transfer to the medical school at Howard University for your final two years."

Howard University is a school set up primarily to open the doors of educational opportunity to blacks as well as whites. Its medical school does not enjoy the reputation of institutions such as Harvard.

McClane, who is black, realized in a few moments that blacks were also included among Hale's many prejudices. Hale's remarks infuriated McClane who stormed out of the interview. As with myself, McClane did not submit his application to Harvard and was able to prove that as a graduate of Boston University he could bring honor on himself and to his community.

Art Wein, another of my medical classmates, revealed some of the prejudices that existed during those years of struggle to be accepted into medical school. He had applied to one of the top schools in Pennsylvania where a physician friend and a strong supporter of that school had written a letter endorsing his application. It was a shocker for his close family friend when a disheartening response was received.

"Thank you for the letter recommending Mr. Wein. Unfortunately, we have already accepted two Jewish students for the coming year. This is our maximum quota, but if Mr. Wein wishes to submit an application next year, we will be glad to consider him."

Such outright open prejudice is not encountered at the present time, but years ago as these examples demonstrate it was not unusual.

Lewis Thomas did not decide on a career in medicine until his last year at Princeton. In his book, "The Youngest Science," he writes that his father, a graduate of Harvard Medical School, had just about given up hopes that his son would ever set his sights on any goal.

During his first three years at college, Thomas revealed that his grades were terrible and he did not apply himself to anything specific. In the last year of school his grades improved and with the encouragement of his father he applied to Harvard. His father was a classmate of Hans Zinsser, the Dean of Harvard Medical School, and world-renowned author. He interviewed young Thomas and agreed that the overall grades did not meet the standards of other applicants. In deference to his father, he recommended Lewis Thomas' admission.

Unquestionably, Worth Hale was bypassed when Lewis Thomas submitted his application, otherwise he too would have been rejected.

Thomas was an outstanding student at Harvard, becoming internationally known for his research and writings on biology, including the best-selling book, "Life of a cell."

Howard P. House became widely accepted for his advanced surgical developments in diseases of the ear during his 50 years of practice. His book, "For the World to Hear," has Ben acclaimed by Ronald Regan, Bob Hope, Norman Vincent Peale, and many others whose hearing he was able to improve .

Dr. House recalls a meeting of the admissions committee of the USC Medical School. In his capacity as chairman, he had submitted the application of an unnamed young man whose marks in his first three years of college were filled with Cs, Ds, and a few Fs. He improved in the fourth year but his average was 2.2, well below the 3.0 required for consideration.

Howard House turned to the other members of the committee and said, "I would like to have you give this student serious consideration."

His statement was greeted with laughter.

One member replied, "Howard, you can't be serious."

The rest of the committee agreed that the application should be rejected.It was then that Dr. House revealed the transcript was his own and had been submitted to USC some 30 years earlier. He related that in his final year of college he had improved his grades but not sufficiently to reach the magic level of 3.0 His interview with a compassionate dean of admissions and strong recommendations turned the tide in his favor.

During many years on the admissions committee at USC, Howard House waged almost a one-man campaign that acceptance into medical school should depend heavily on a personal interview and supportive letters rather than scholastic records alone. From my own experience, I agree with him wholeheartedly.

Boston University must rank near the top for opening its doors to all groups no matter what their sex or ethnic background might be. At one of our reunions I noted that my classmates included Greek, Lithuanian, Polish, Italian, Irish, and Jewish parentage as well as Ken McClane who I mentioned before is black. There were three women in our freshman class but they dropped out before graduation due to marriage and pregnancy.

During a recent visit to BU Medical, I had a conversation with a student of the junior class. She revealed that just under 50% of the members were women. It may not be true in the upper echelons of the business world but in medicine, especially BU, women are well represented.

A few years ago a young man wrote a letter published in the New England Journal of Medicine. He complained that despite his desire to gain a medical degree, become a pediatrician, and take care of impoverished children, he had turned down his acceptance to medical school.

He lamented that his training program would entail many years of expense that would be a financial burden and take a lifetime to completely resolve. Apparently, despite his protestations, the word sacrifice was not in this young man's vocabulary.

I have quoted aphorisms of my mother quite frequently. A favorite of hers was "Where there is a will, there is a way." This was true when we were growing up and continues to be the pathway to success for many young people today.

Private and government organizations have now made it possible for aspiring students to enter the medical field. They may require a commitment to several years of service in poverty-stricken parts of the country and the world. The opportunities for the truly dedicated are without limits.

"I am Going to Die"

While pushing through the half-open door I could hear the groaning sounds and mumbling of the patient who was one of my assignments on

District Medicine that morning. I approached the bed near the window and saw the unshaven face of an elderly male peering out from the torn blankets that partially covered his body.

With a fearful, frightened expression, he greeted me with a statement of impending doom.

"*Doctor!* I am going to die. I am going to die."

As a third-year student at Boston University Medical School, one month included seeing patients in their homes located in the neighborhood. During this period, the students met each morning at 8 AM in the Outpatient Department of the Boston City Hospital. Our guidance instructor passed out the assignments for each student.

Some of the patients on our lists were follow-up cases for routine examination. Others were new individuals who were apparently not severely ill. If the call seemed like an emergency, an ambulance was dispatched immediately for the patient's admission.

The area covered by the students was no more than a half mile from the hospital which, in those days, was a 2000-bed institution. The Boston City Hospital had become world renowned for its research on anemias, burn treatments, and many other therapies. It was a desirable place to find the answers to the perplexing questions that faced the practicing physician and the young medical student.

The home I visited that morning was rather typical of the surroundings. Practically all were rooming houses, dilapidated apartments, or rodent-infested, rundown hotels. Yet during my entire month on service I never once encountered nor heard of any muggings or attempted assaults. Most of the patients were in the older age group and lived alone. There were some young mothers with children, some widowed or divorced, and of course the single mother with children but no visible father.

The usual routine during the weeks of service included examination of the patient and the prescribing of a single medication that might be indicated. Suggestions for diet were made where practical as well as recommendations to improve the personal sanitation of the individual.

This sixty-year-old pale, prematurely aged white male was obviously apprehensive and concerned. I tried to reassure him during the examination, telling him that he was not about to die, but he just continued to repeat the same words over and over again, "I am going to die. I am going to die."

During our limited exposure to sick people in the medical clinics and district medicine, we had seen several patients who expressed a fear of dying. There is an old Scotch proverb that states "There is no medicine for fear," and this is especially true for those who live alone. No matter how minimal their symptoms, it is the specter of dying alone and not death that fills them with anguish.

While examining the patient, I truly felt that his premonition of death was exaggerated. He complained of slight pressure in his chest and although his color was pale, he did not have the ashen or gray facies that one would expect to find in a patient who is about to die.

"Your pulse and blood pressure are really not too bad. I don't think that you are going to die. Let me give you some medicine that will make you comfortable and tomorrow I will come back and check you again."

Since my examination proved to be essentially negative, it appeared to me that he probably had a mild anginal attack causing his chest pain aggravated by his apprehension. I was sure the nitroglycerine tablets that I was going to give him would take care of his problem. Despite my words of encouragement, he kept repeating again and again, "I am going to die. I am going to die."

After listening to his anguished tones and forebodings I decided that under the circumstances his judgment was better than mine. I made arrangements for him to be seen in the emergency room. Before leaving the patient I again reassured him that he had no cause for concern and that I would check him again after his admission to the hospital.

He was my last visit of the morning and after making the phone call to the hospital for his admission, I walked back to the hospital cafeteria for lunch. After that I checked on my patient's status in the emergency room.

It was a real shock when I was directed to the section for the critically ill. Pulling the curtain back from his assigned bed, I discovered that my patient was in the process of being pronounced dead. He had been admitted about a half hour earlier and died a few minutes before my arrival. An autopsy later that afternoon revealed that he had suffered a heart attack.

When reviewing the case with the instructor, he reassured me that my evaluation had been correct.

"There was no reason to suspect a serious heart problem in view of your examination. You had no access to an EKG which could have identified the problem. More importantly was your decision to admit the patient to the hospital although even that could not save his life."

I did learn a valuable lesson that was never forgotten. Always listen to the patient and when they say they are going to die, give them reassurance, but be prepared for the inevitable. It is true that many patients exaggerate their symptoms, but the doctor must use his best judgment in his evaluation.

In modern medicine there is a tendency to utilize all the technological advantages at our disposal. This may be influenced at times by the threat of malpractice, but it does increase the cost of medical care. Very often a careful evaluation of the patient by the physician will relieve the victim of their concern and quite often the symptoms. If there is continued apprehension it might be best to believe the individual and arrange for admission to the hospital.

More and more as we scan the news we read about some patient who had been turned away from the emergency room as having no disease. Later the distraught family reveals that the ill victim died several hours after returning from the hospital. Medicine is not an exact science and honest mistakes can occur, but doctors will become more suspect when a judgement mistake happens.

My decision to arrange for the patient's admission to the hospital was due more to a sense of compassion for the patient than my limited medical knowledge. I tried to maintain this type of empathy for patients during my years of active practice. The vast majority of physicians with whom I have been associated have always exhibited this same ability to understand, to be sensitive to, and to experience vicariously the feelings of our patients. Unfortunately, in this increasingly materialistic world there are a number of physicians who do not share this feeling of consideration and the patients are the losers.

Who Killed Beano Breen?

"Beano Breen Dies Despite Heroic Efforts of Surgeons."

When I read this headline and the reports of the shooting of Beano Breen in the newspaper, my thoughts went back to the sequence of events early that morning.

It was just after midnight and I had turned out the light, hoping for an uninterrupted sleep. The phone rang and being the only medical student in the room that night the call obviously had to be for me. I walked over to the far side of the room and picked up the phone. I heard the familiar voice of Moe, the senior surgical resident.

"Curran, there's an accident case in the emergency room. Go down and check on it. If you need any help, call me."

As a third-year Boston University medical student, I was able to convince Dr. Louis Schwartz that I could do a good job as a sub-junior interne at the Boston City Hospital. Dr. Schwartz, an assistant administrator, had multiple responsibilities, among them being the assignment of two medical students from Tufts, Harvard, and Boston University to act as night assistants in their school's medical or surgical department during the junior year.

The appointment to BU's surgical section gave me a bed in the large dormitory room on the top floor of the internes' building and access to free meals in the hospital cafeteria. The duties of the six students included simple laboratory procedures such as blood counts and urine examinations, as well as starting transfusions and intravenous fluids. An added bonus in my assignment was the chance to assist at surgery and on occasion, to give the anesthetic under the supervision of the anesthesia resident.

In the emergency room we were often allowed to sew up lacerations. One way or another we were always on the scene as the drama of life and death took place while hundreds of patients streamed through the hospital doors every hour of the day and night. Despite this, some of our group considered themselves as glorified gofers, "Go for this or go for that." To others, it was just "scut" work, just one step above an orderly level. But to me it was a glorious opportunity to see and work in an atmosphere probably unequaled in any other hospital in the country.

When Moe called that night his form of address was quite typical. He was not the kind of person who might say "would you?" or "please." It was not that, as sub-juniors, we expected to be addressed in any special manner, but most of the other internes and residents whom we met were pleasant, sociable, and generally respectful.

I got along with Moe, but would never think of crossing him in any way. First, because of his size, six-foot-four and weighing about 250 pounds. He also had a noticeable lack of polish and a brusque, almost hostile manner. His general appearance was not especially attractive since he was rarely clean shaven and often looked as if he had slept in his clothes. Not many of the personnel had a kind word for him, but I followed him around like a puppy dog. There was much to learn at this huge hospital and I was willing to crawl if necessary to find all the answers.

After receiving Moe's call I wasted no time getting to the emergency room where the nursing supervisor directed me to the location of the patient. That proved to be an obstacle course, since his stretcher was surrounded by a nurse, two orderlies, and two men dressed in street clothes. The latter two, I learned, were detectives from police headquarters.

The history, taken by the admitting doctor, stated that the patient had been shot behind the left ear. The victim's name was Beano Breen, which meant nothing to me at the time. He was a stocky man in his early fifties, just under six-feet-tall and weighing about 200 pounds. He had a broad barrel chest and a short thick neck. I found out later he had been a professional boxer in his youth.

The routine examination, including the heart and lungs, was negative. I removed the bandage that had been placed behind his left ear by the admitting physician. A small slightly irregular round hole covered by dry blood was the only sign of injury.

"You have been shot," I said, leaning over close to the patient.

I tried to sound very authoritative, but the patient, who was awake and alert, indicated by his manner that he was not at all impressed by me. Despite my doctor's garb, Beano gave me no more response than he would show an orderly. The only reaction I received was a furtive glance over my shoulder at the two detectives standing behind me. They were obviously waiting for the victim to give some information as to "who did the shooting or whom he suspected."

Although he was fully conscious, Beano gave no indication that he was about to talk. He was following a typical gangster's code as I later realized. Edward G. Robinson or George Raft, well-known movie stars of hoodlum roles in that era, would have carried off Beano's part to perfection.

I called Moe.

"There's a man down here," I said, "who has been shot and is conscious, but not talking. What do you want me to do?"

Moe's response was immediate.

"I'll be right down," he snapped.

During my short period of duty on the surgical service, I had learned that there is a certain amount of appeal to house officers when a shooting occurs. It helps to break up the monotony of the routine case work which is so much a part of the resident's duties. They liked the action and in a big city hospital such as the BCH, they would frequently get it.

After Moe's arrival he quickly ordered some x-ray studies and then hastily reviewed them. Along with some of his other failings, he tended to be rather impetuous. Coming back to the patient he announced that the patient needed to be explored immediately so that the bullet could be removed.

The x-rays clearly revealed the metallic outline of the bullet in the tissues of the neck just below the left ear. It looked like a simple case, but in view of the circumstances, I thought Moe should at least contact the attending surgical chief. Usually permission for surgery is obtained, but this resident did not always follow protocol and did not do so in this case.

"Curran," he said, "we are going to take the patient into the minor surgical room and remove the bullet. Do you know how to give Evipal?"

"Yes," I answered quickly. "I have given that anesthetic a number of times while working with Dr. Marcus, the anesthesia resident."

Beano Breen was quickly wheeled into the room that was set up for surgery where I helped strap him to the surgical stretcher. All this time Beano lay back quietly, only his eyes moving from one person to the next, perhaps in wonderment, but not one word escaping from his lips.

Moe casually mentioned to the patient that the bullet was going to be removed. There were no other words of explanation by Moe and no questions from Beano.

While Moe checked over the instruments laid out for the surgery, I gathered the equipment needed to put the patient to sleep. After prepping the right arm with an alcohol sponge, I identified the vein to be used for injection of the anesthetic.

Having spent many hours the previous year taking blood from patients at the hospital's syphilis clinic, I knew that getting the needle into a vein would not be a problem. While Moe scrubbed for the surgery, I put the tourniquet on the patient's arm and prepared to insert the needle into the vein. I felt confident and important in being part of the team.

Suddenly I felt a firm brush from behind. It was Moe who had stopped scrubbing, having decided to give the anesthetic himself. The syringe of Evipal was literally torn from my hands as Moe quickly palpated the same vein that I was about to use for the injection.

During the short period of time that Evipal had been used in the United States there had been a number of fatalities reported. One of the problems was the sudden development of laryngospasm (spasmodic closure of the larynx) that could occur shortly after it was administered, especially if the injection was not given slowly. When this took place the patient developed severe difficulty in breathing with a generalized muscle spasm as the patient desperately fought for air. It was several years before a similar but safer anesthetic, Pentothal, was developed. Unfortunately, it too could precipitate laryngospasm in some patients.

As Moe pushed me aside and took over, I reluctantly stood by feeling that I had been denied an opportunity to be an essential part of the operating team. In a few moments, however, I quickly forgot my chagrin at not being allowed to give the intravenous anesthetic.

Moe quickly inserted the needle into the vein and pumped the syringeful of Evipal with one rapid motion. Beano Breen gasped and his face became florid as laryngospasm developed immediately. I hadn't seen this occur when using the anesthetic under the guidance of Dr. Marcus, although he assured me that it could happen with any patient, especially if the Evipal is injected very quickly.

When spasmodic closure of the larynx occurs, no oxygen is available to the patient and breathing is severely impeded and frequently stops completely.

Although Moe had stopped injecting the Evipal, Beano Breen's spasms increased. The intense ruddy color of his face and neck became replaced by extreme pallor and then a bluish hue. The veins of his neck were now distended and his eyes bulged.

Suddenly Beano began vomiting as his whole body convulsed in a massive seizure. He shook violently on the stretcher as his lungs were gasping for air, but the larynx was shut down tight from the effects of the Evipal.

Apparently Beano Breen had consumed a meal of spaghetti just prior to being shot. His stomach contents erupted forcefully, filling his mouth and throat with the vomitus which was then sucked down into the windpipe, plugging off the airway completely.

Suddenly his body stopped moving and panic took over as Moe with his huge arms pressed on the chest in a vain attempt to start Beano's breathing again. In the meantime I furiously suctioned his mouth, trying to clear the airway by removing the globs of spaghetti which had filled his throat.

While Moe continued to press rhythmically on Beano's chest, grunting all the while, I snapped a stethoscope onto my ears hoping to pick up the sound of a heart beat. All I could hear was the swishing sound of the chest movement as Moe continued his efforts to get air into the lungs. In a few moments, Dr. Marcus, the anesthesia resident arrived to continue the resuscitation efforts, but it was futile. Beano Breen was dead.

As they wheeled the stretcher bearing the patient's body toward the autopsy room, Dr. Marcus explained what had happened to cause the tragedy.

"First," he said, "the patient had the barrel-type chest and short neck that made him much more susceptible to laryngospasm with any anesthetic, especially Evipal. Additionally, he had recently eaten a big meal which dramatically increases his risk. With his projectile vomiting, the food got into his throat stimulating the gag reflex, causing the material to be aspirated into the windpipe and lungs."

Marcus gave me one more word of caution which I already knew, but now it was more dramatic in view of the events that had transpired.

"Never, never," he said, "give this intravenous anesthetic quickly since it can be a sure path to disaster."

While walking back to my room, I thought how close I had come to being the one who pushed the fatal anesthetic into the victim's bloodstream. I don't know if it bothered Moe since I never asked. It served to remind me not to take on any procedure without solid knowledge of all the complications that might develop.

The autopsy report issued later that morning stated that a bullet was found in the tissues of the neck close to the carotid artery, a major blood vessel leading to the brain. Death was due to asphyxiation caused by aspiration of food, identified as spaghetti, into the lungs. The artery showed no evidence of injury.

A few days after the death of Beano Breen, I met Dr. Joe Corcoran, the admitting physician when Breen was first brought to the Boston City Hospital. Dr. Corcoran's description of his involvement was fascinating and indeed, almost bizarre.

"I saw the patient when he had been taken by taxicab to the emergency room after being shot in the Metropolitan Hotel lobby. Several shots were said to have been fired, but I only found a small bullet hole behind his left ear. After covering the wound with a small dressing, I asked the supervisor to contact the 4th surgical service which was responsible for the care of the next emergency."

Revealing my part in the case, I said, "That's when Moe called me."

Corcoran continued, "I heard that Breen had choked on a cigar."

He was amazed when I told him that the patient had been prepared for surgery and died after the injection of the Evipal anesthesia.

Dr. Corcoran added, "Knowing Moe, I am not surprised at what he did."

Joe Corcoran then revealed an amazing twist of events that took place after the death of Beano Breen.

"About 2 AM," he said, "after the patient had expired, I received a phone call asking me to see Joe Guaragna the night superintendent immediately."

Corcoran's strange story continued:

"I went to Guaragna's office which is located off the main floor of the emergency area, as you know. Coming toward me were two typical north-end characters, obviously of Italian and probably of Sicilian extraction. Instead of allowing me to pass, they blocked my way so that I couldn't enter the superintendent's office. The more sinister of the two in a dark suit, black shirt, white silk tie, and a black fedora pulled down over his eyes, grabbed the front of my hospital jacket. He pinned me against the wall and barked, 'You, Corcoran. You da Doc dat took care of Beano Breen up front?' 'That's right,' I said. 'What's the problem?' 'His wallet, his dough, and da diamond watch. Da diamond stickpin, too.' I was completely mystified for a moment. 'Oh, that stuff,' I said. 'The orderlies who undressed him put his clothes and all his belongings in a hospital bag and took it to the admitting clerk to be locked up.' The response to that was a threatening grunt, 'Don't gimme no crap! The clerk says he aint seen no dough and no jewelry. Just da clothes. Dat watch was worth five grand and Beano always carried plenty cash.'"

Joe Corcoran admitted that he was worried.

"Still wondering what was going to happen to me next, the two of them pushed me ahead toward Joe Guaragna's office. Once in the office, the squinty-eyed leader asked the superintendent, 'Is dis da jerk you said worked on Beano and he didn't send you no watch and no dough, right?' I was dumbfounded when Guaragna replied, 'All I got was a bag of clothes, no watch and no money, like I told you before.'"

Corcoran said he became really upset when the smaller thug grabbed him yelling, "Give!"

But then Joe Guaragna burst out laughing and introduced him to the two gangsters. The one doing most of the yelling was an assistant district attorney and the other was one of his investigators who happened to be Guaragna's cousin.

As Joe Corcoran recalled, "They all enjoyed a good laugh at my expense and revealed that the superintendent had put them up to the gag."

Dr. Corcoran's description of the events surrounding Beano Breen's death became even more incredible when the newspaper stories developed two days later. It was established that Breen had been robbed of his wallet, watch, and diamond stickpin by one of the accident-floor orderlies. This employee confessed to the robbery and surrendered the stolen articles.

The arrest, trial, and conviction of the orderly, with his subsequent sentencing to the Charles Street jail resulted in many newspaper articles. For a short while this proved to be a tremendous source of embarrassment to Dr. Corcoran and his family. Many friends and acquaintances around Boston knew that he worked at the Boston City Hospital Emergency Room as an admitting physician. They called to offer their condolences to him and his family. One attorney even volunteered free legal help.

By an amazing coincidence the orderly, who went to prison for the robbery, worked the night shift. He was about the same age and his name happened to be John Joseph Corcoran, exactly the same as Dr. Corcoran. This namesake orderly was the ringleader of the hospital personnel who were involved in Beano Breen's robbery.

All of this led to a full-blown investigation which revealed the extent of pilfering that was taking place at the hospital. Accident victims especially had often been admitted in an unconscious state along with drunks who were frequently brought to the hospital in a stuporous condition. Neither the drunks nor the accident victims found a listening ear when they complained that money and other valuables had been taken from their clothing. The appeals from families of dying patients were ignored when they mentioned such losses. It was not until Beano Breen also became a victim of this ghoulish practice that the authorities took positive action.

For several weeks after Breen's death, the Boston newspapers filled their pages with stories about his longtime legal encounters. According to the Boston Globe, he had been arrested 35 times, but never spent a day in jail. He had been suspected of involvement in at least two murders and many assault charges had been filed against him with no convictions. He used his fists as he had done in his boxing career to settle many of his arguments.

A reporter for the Boston Post wrote that Breen had been contacted by a gang leader to help put a Revere dry-cleaning establishment out of business. The gangster had been hired by the union that had been carrying on a strike against the company for some months. Beano apparently agreed to do the gangster's bidding for a hefty consideration, but then came the double cross.

Beano also took $20,000 from the dry-cleaning owner to keep his business from being wrecked. To further complicate the whole scenario, it was also revealed that Breen was trying to chisel in on the numbers-pool play that was such a profitable source of income to the mob. There was no doubt that those mobsters had put Breen on their hit list. The assailant who shot Breen was never identified although a number of suspects were interrogated.

The question may be asked: What caused Beano Breen's death? Was it an assassin's bullet or was the cause iatrogenic, i.e. resulting from the surgical resident's anesthetic injection? Again we have only the coroner's report which was signed out as "Death due to asphyxiation secondary to aspiration of food, spaghetti."

Surviving Financially as a Medical Student

Working evenings as a drugstore clerk, greasing New Haven Railroad engines, or doing road construction during the summer eased my financial burdens before medical school. The extra hours of clinical duties in my third year at Boston University Medical School eliminated any chance of night work at the store. However, the appointment as a sub-junior interne at the Boston City Hospital assured me of bed and board for that junior year.

In addition to this experience with BU surgical service, the student interneship brought me in close contact with the resident assigned to the 4th surgical service. Frequently, an emergency operation required type O blood and almost on a regular monthly basis, I would be called as a donor. The $25.00 fee received took care of my expenses which were pretty minimal.

The engagement of my sister to George McGunnigle, a theater manager, guaranteed passes to a movie every few weeks. The free esplanade concerts and the theater were within a mile of the City Hospital. A lovely, redheaded student nurse, Mary Earley, was in training at the hospital and with no car for transportation, we walked to our entertainment destinations. The only expense was Brigham's ice cream shop where soda cost fifteen cents. Mary's class was described as "angels in white travelling along the corridors of death spreading their works of mercy."

Strolling hand in hand gave little chance for romance, but much conversation about the events of the day and our thoughts and dreams of the future.

Blood Money Saves my Specialty Training

The money received for giving transfusions caused me no apparent difficulties until the end of my junior year in 1938. At that time the drums of war were beating in Europe as Hitler embarked on his ill-fated attempt to take over all the countries in Europe. It was clear that the United States was building up the armed forces prior to entering the conflict. Many rumors floated about that if the medical students did not sign up for the reserves they would be inducted as buck privates. I never heard of this ever taking place, but most of the class decided to join up.

Several of my classmates were not too enthused about a commitment to the service before graduation. Jack Davis and I became close friends since we had been seated alphabetically from our first year in medical school.

I asked Jack, who was very astute, what he planned on doing. After some hesitation, he replied, "Frankly, I am not too sure what to do. If we join now we may be put into the army immediately and have no choice as to where we will go. However, by waiting until we finish school we may have a better idea as to what branch of service is best for us."

"That's right, Jack," I said. "But if the stories we hear are correct we might end up as privates or find ourselves overseas as infantry doctors."

After further discussion, I decided that it was best to join the crowd and arrange for my physical examination. Who knows what the future is likely to bring?

As I said to Jack, "Members of the reserve will be compensated for attending meetings in our last year of school and during the one year of our interneship. That is something that I can use."

Along with several other classmates a date was set up for the physical examination at the armory located a short distance from the medical school. A day before the scheduled exam I was called to give a pint of blood for a surgical patient. The request came from Dr. Connor.

He said, "This patient has a bleeding ulcer and is having surgery today. We need the blood before the operation."

"Dr. Connor," I said. "I would like to give the blood, but I gave a pint just one week ago. Do you think giving another pint this soon might be risky for me?"

"You should have no problem," Dr. Connor said. "The patient needs the blood desperately, but I will only take a half pint and see that you are reimbursed with the full $25.00 payment."

That was a deal I could not refuse. The blood was duly taken and there were no noticeable side effects.

About an hour before heading for the army physical I spoke to Jack Davis.

"Even though I feel OK, Jack," I said, "would you please check my blood pressure? That extra blood I gave yesterday may have caused some changes."

After taking a reading, Jack pulled back in surprise.

"Your pressure is only 80/60, Tim," he said. "You can't possibly pass the exam with that low reading."

"Take another reading, Jack," I said. The subnormal BP was beginning to worry me.

The subsequent pressures taken by Jack showed no change. They were all low in the same range as the first reading. My blood pressure in the past had never varied from the normal, usually around 120/70. There was only one thing to do and that was to call the armory and cancel the physical.

I never did decide on another physical for the army reserves although my blood pressure reading repeated some weeks later had returned to normal. The majority of my classmates who were examined in their junior year were inducted into the service after finishing their one year of interneship. This resulted in an assignment to general medicine duty followed by service with combat infantry forces.

The completion of my ENT training was especially helpful in treating the multiple ear and sinus complaints of air force personnel who became my responsibility.

3

INTERNESHIP

Where to Interne?

"Where are you going to interne?"

In our class of some 75 seniors, this became a common topic of conversation. Interneship following graduation from medical school lasted one year and was a preparation for general practice and also a prerequisite for more advanced training in the various specialities.

Prior to making formal application for interneship, I met a friend who graduated from BU and took his interneship at St. Francis Hospital in Hartford, Connecticut, just 100 miles from Boston. Being a rather provincial individual, I didn't want to stray too far from my home base. I wanted to to be close to my family and Mary Earley, the student nurse at the Boston City Hospital. Frankly, I was smitten by her, but financially at this stage in our lives there was no way that marriage could be considered.

My friend, Tom Feeney, helped me to make my decision about where to interne.

"St. Francis has a top-notch staff with excellent facilities. In addition, they pay $10.00 a month and the food is excellent."

Inquiries regarding other hospitals in New England indicated that in most cases there was absolutely no monetary compensation. Additionally, many of the reports indicated that although the interne staff did not suffer from malnutrition, the food left much to be desired.

After visiting several comparable hospitals within commuting distance by bus or train, I decided on St. Francis Hospital and never regretted my decision.

There were relatively few minor problems that were irksome to our group of ten internes. One major advantage was having our own separate quarters on the hospital grounds.

This had been the home and the first hospital for eight patients and a brave little company of six nuns. They were enticed to leave their homeland in France with dreams of a magnificent medical facility. Their initial disappointment on arrival in 1897 was turned eventually into the

29

reality of a modern hospital. Their venture succeeded only through the endeavors and steadfastness of their administrator, Mother Valencia, who had accompanied them from their convent in France. She overcame the animosity of the neighbors and won the support of the legislature for approval of what became a leading medical institution. Her inability to speak fluent English failed to be an impediment as she guided the successful progress of the hospital.

The nuns who occupied the original small building, now the internes' quarters, would probably turn over in their graves if they became witnesses to the activities that had become part of the daily life of the young doctors who occupied their former home.

The internes were not overly destructive, but at times especially on weekends, they were a bit exuberant. On one occasion, the partying became rougher than usual and ended with a few broken chairs, a surplus of empty beer bottles and cans, and a general mess. The housekeeper complained to the administrator, Mother Xavier, who had succeeded Mother Valencia. The penalty was forfeiture of our $10.00 monthly stipend. There were no interne demands or threats of striking and of course, no picketing or slowdown of our daily duties. We meekly accepted our penalty and became a little less rambunctious in our future social affairs.

Looking back on our training period, it might seem that our interneship was a year of slave labor, especially in comparison with present day standards. However, we accepted those twelve months as a time to be instructed not just from the textbook, but in the care of patients in our everyday practice.

The young men and women who are being trained in hospitals are now receiving the just compensation they deserve. Our generation, although receiving minimal financial rewards during training, did not suffer in those lean years. Once they began practice their income was adequate to raise a family and live in a pleasant middle-class neighborhood. Those of us who had their careers in medicine delayed by military service regretted the delay, but were thankful that we returned to civilian life without a disabling injury. I was fortunate in being accepted on the staff of the hospital where I served my interneship and established lifelong associations and friendships.

An Interne's Day and Night

The duties of the internes covered a broad spectrum of assignments, starting with daily rounds at 7 AM. The attending physician would review the private and ward cases which were his responsibility and we had an opportunity to question the treatment he recommended and offer alternatives.

As an interne on the surgical service, it was expected that we would assist on operative procedures. That required us to be finished with rounds and scrubbed and gowned in the operating room ready to start at the appointed time of 8 o'clock.

The modern hospital has a full array of technicians who cover many facets of hospital care that were once the responsibility of the interne staff. Although the laboratory technicians performed routine tests during the day, the interne had to be prepared to do many of these examinations if ordered in the evening. The taking of blood samples, administering blood transfusions, and other intravenous fluids were also included in our daily routine.

During the daily rounds one interne was irked by an older physician who greeted him and other internes one morning.

"How are all the juveniles today?"

"Fine, how are all the seniles?" the interne answered.

The staff physician was not considered very sharp medically and tended to be overly critical of the interne staff. The interne's response was not proper, but understandable under the circumstances.

Duty scheduling was arranged so that alternate nights and weekends were free. Holidays were also arranged by common agreement so that each interne, by lot or choice, worked equal time for such events. If an interne had call duty at night he was expected to be available at the usual time the next morning even though he may have been busy the entire night. I never knew of anyone who failed to show up or collapsed after a full night of emergency calls, but there were some days when we were pretty lethargic.

A Missed Diagnosis or Was It?

"Diagnosis: Gastroenteritis. Treatment: Better food."

When I wrote those notes on the patient's chart I should have known that it was going to cause me some trouble.

My one-year service of internship included two months on internal medicine. One morning the request came to check a student nurse who was admitted with severe stomach pains.

The young lady had a typical history of gastroenteritis.

"I woke up during the night with stomach cramps and then diarrhea," she said.

"Do you get these symptoms often?"

"No. I don't recall ever being sick like this before."

"What did you have for your evening meal?" I asked.

"The same as all the other nurses, frankfurts and beans."

The physical exam was unremarkable except for some general tenderness over her abdomen. A blood count and urinanalysis had been done before I saw the young lady and the results were all within normal limits. Her temperature was a half degree above normal which was not significant.

After finishing the examination and reviewing the history, there was no doubt in my mind that the student nurse had a severe attack of gastroenteritis. The internes and the student nurses had been served the same food the night before. Some of us, including myself, experienced mild stomach cramps and diarrhea. My patient's symptoms of acute and severe discomfort suggested the need for hospitalization for observation.

I completed my evaluation and wrote down the diagnosis, recommending an anti-diarrheal medication and the forcing of fluids. My additional suggestion of a better quality of food was totally uncalled for, although I thought that might alert the dietitian that something was not quite right.

The nurse in charge of the ward, Sister Mary Edwards, did not take kindly to my semihumorous remark or diagnosis. She called in a surgeon who was on service at the time. The interne staff did not have much respect for this doctor as a surgeon or as a diagnostician. He decided that the patient had acute appendicitis requiring immediate surgery. I was crushed by his decision since I felt that my diagnosis, if not the recommended treatment, was correct.

After the surgery had been performed, Sister Edwards brought the chart to the attention of the administrator. She notified Dr. James of my transgression and demanded that he take some action. According to Dr. James, "she was really upset."

A few days later, I was approached by the Chairman of the Interne Committee, Dr. Lewis James himself, a very competent and respected member of the obstetrical staff. He had a simple request: "Would you please change your diagnosis and your suggested treatment?"

I changed the treatment suggesting better food, but I was still annoyed about the decision which precipitated the surgery. Another opinion, I believed, could have avoided surgical intervention.

Later I checked with Gerry Mitchell, a friend of mine, who was serving as a resident in the department of pathology.

"Tell me, Gerry, was that really an acute appendix that was removed from the student nurse?"

Gerry's answer was immediate.

"It was a worm," he said.

This was a common pathology term for an appendix that after removal showed no evidence of disease or acute infection.

It made me feel better, but I did regret not being more professional and discreet in reporting my findings and my recommendations. I had also been forced to make a change in the chart by rewriting my report. As an interne making that revision, I avoided further penalties from the administration. Any practicing physician who makes such revisions in his records could find himself in some legal trouble.

My Last Day as an Obstetrician

The month of obstetrics during my year of interneship was coming to a close. It had been enjoyable and interesting, but delivering babies mostly at night would not be my first choice for a future medical practice.

My last night on call was interrupted sometime after the the hour of midnight. Being the obstetrical interne required spending the night in a room next to the delivery area. Frequently the expectant mother delayed her departure to the hospital or the baby was impatient for its entry into the world. For these reasons it was not uncommon for a precipitate delivery to occur shortly after the mother reached the hospital.

There was not much time wasted in this child's arrival. Even though I was in the delivery room moments after being awakened, the nurses were ready to take over my duties by the time I reached the mother's side. In most cases birth can take place without doctors or nurses, but it is recognized that in such situations the complication rate rises. Having an available interne serving as an obstetrician is an added safeguard for the mother and baby

If the attending physician is not immediately available for his private patients, the interne becomes the obstetrician of record and signs the sheet accordingly. This particular mother was being followed regularly in the obstetrical clinic, although it happened that I had not seen her on any of the days I was on duty.

The mother and the baby came through the delivery without complication and I checked them each day until they left the hospital four days later. At that time I noted that this was the patient's third child, all born out of wedlock. Without attempting to sermonize, but feebly trying to give some helpful advice, I spent a few minutes with her prior to her discharge. I gently reminded her that she had now given birth to three children with no apparent identity of the father.

"Mandy," I said, "why don't you get married and enjoy a home with a father for these children. He could help you take care of them and also give you some attention."

Her response was quick and positive.

"Doctor," she said with wickedness flashing in her eyes, "why should I make one man miserable when I am making so many men happy?"

I thought her answer was succinct and to the point. When I mentioned the conversation to the nun in charge, she was not impressed by my advice or the mother's response.

Some years after starting practice, I had occasion to stop at the hospital admissions office. A young lady just recently hired, introduced herself to me and then turned to another secretary and said that I was her mother's obstetrician.

"I'm sorry," I said. "You must have me mixed up with another physician. My specialty is ear, nose, and throat."

She insisted that she was right.

"I'll bring in the birth certificate and prove it," she said emphatically.

The next morning, while walking by her office, she stopped me and waved a paper in front of my face. Sure enough, there was my name affixed to the birth certificate with the date of the month I was on service.

I don't know how many private patients I delivered during that period, but I do recall that there were at least a half dozen mothers whose delivery was precipitous and the private physician was not immediately available, thus making me the responsible physician and the obstetrician of record. The young lady beamed as she watched the surprised look on my face. She made a copy of the certificate which I proudly placed on the wall of my office along with my diplomas and other citations.

Choosing otolaryngology instead of obstetrics was a decision I never regretted, but I can appreciate the affection that most women have for their obstetricians who helped to make their lives more complete. It seems so unfair and unfortunate that in this day of skyrocketing medical malpractice premiums, the delivery of babies brings on the greatest number of suits and consequently the highest insurance costs. It has caused a great number of honest and capable physicians to retire from this specialty. Many malpractice actions are justified, but it would often take the wisdom of a King Solomon to render a just decision when an unexpected mishap occurs during a delivery of a newborn.

On Call New Year's Eve
A Near Disaster

Being the interne on duty for New Year's Eve proved to be uneventful until late that night when a call came to check on several patients. Included in the calls was a request from one doctor who asked that a blood count and urine be done on his patient who was complaining of stomach cramps. An examination of the patient and a quick history indicated nothing of significance. The blood and urine samples were taken, but I decided that the report, being obviously negative, should be deferred to a later hour.

After completing the lab work, I decided to drop by and say hello to Jack McCarthy, a patient whom I first met during my month on neurosurgery. Despite being paralyzed from the waist down and confined to his bed and wheelchair, he never complained about his disability or the pain he suffered. He was a great reader and knowledgeable about many things with a keen interest in politics.

Coming from Boston and being involved in the political scene because of my brother John's interest in the Democratic party, I was also a mildly vocal supporter of Jim Curley, many-times mayor of Boston. The admiration of Curley was not shared by a lot of people, especially the Brahmins who had ruled that city for several centuries. There were stories about this well-known politician that described him as a saint or a sinner depending on the narrator. I had heard these tales from my brother and of course read about Curley in the local press which treated him with disdain.

The Telegram, considered the scandal sheet of the Boston press, was an especially harsh critic of Curley. On one occasion the paper's editor, Pelletier, displayed his venom in a full front-page cartoon showing Curley with a ball and chain attached to his legs. It was captioned "Curley the Jailbird" with reference to the occasion many years before when Curley served 30 days in jail after being found guilty of taking a post-office examination for a friend. The next day Curley met Pelletier not too far from City Hall, knocked him down with one blow and proceeded on his way. It established Curley as the Rambo of his day and helped to insure his reelection that year as Mayor of Boston.

It was now 11:30 PM so it seemed like a good time to call the physician who had ordered the laboratory work.

"Dr. Burke," I said in my best professorial tones, lowering my voice an octave, "I have finished the urine examination on Mrs. Walsh and it's completely negative. I will call you later on the results of the blood count."

I could hear Burke sputtering in a sleepy voice as I quickly hung up.

After chatting with Jack McCarthy for another 20 minutes, I dialed Dr. Burke's number again. The phone rang many times before the good doctor answered it in a groggy voice.

"Hello, this is Dr. Burke speaking."

"This is Dr. Curran again with the blood report that you ordered."

"Why the hell are you calling me at this ungodly hour of the night?" he barked.

Now he sounded fully awake.

"Well," I said, "I knew that you were concerned or you would not have requested it as an emergency this evening. I want you to know that the count is completely normal."

The phone was abruptly banged in my ear and I smilingly replaced the receiver. I knew that Dr. Burke would not order another late night laboratory procedure unless it was absolutely indicated.

The evening was now progressing toward midnight. I started to leave and Jack's nurse stopped me.

"Won't you join Jack in a libation to toast the New Year?"

Reluctantly I foolishly agreed, but restricting it only to a glass of ginger ale and maybe a few drops of Canadian whiskey which was resting on the bedside table. My alcohol intake was usually limited to a glass of beer and that was only on rare occasions.

I continued to talk with Jack while the nurse prepared the drinks.

After quickly draining my glass and wondering why the ginger ale burned as it went down, I could hear the sounds of Guy Lombardo playing "Auld Lang Syne" with the bells and cheers from Times Square in the background. Suddenly my own ears started to ring as I experienced an unusual unsteadiness that I had never felt before.

I am sure that it wasn't intentional, but apparently the proportions of whiskey and ginger ale were obviously reversed. Quickly wishing Jack and his nurse a happy New Year, I stepped into the hallway and somehow found myself facing the room used by the administrator as her sleeping quarters.

Loudly banging on her door, I now sent my holiday greetings to Mother Xavier. Before my salutation could be acknowledged by the administrator, whom I could hear shuffling about in her room, I was rescued by Mary Caldwell, the night nursing supervisor. With a forceful hand on my jacket, she pulled and half-dragged me into the elevator and headed me toward the interne's quarters where I collapsed on my bed.

I never did discover if Mother Xavier suspected me as the culprit who knocked on her door, but I'm sure that Mary, always a great friend, saved me from expulsion as an interne. Most of the nuns had a good sense of humor, but our administrator was not one of them especially in a situation such as this.

4

Residency Training

$0 a Month

Ear, nose, and throat residencies after one year of interneship were difficult to obtain in the 1940s. Being a Bostonian, my first thought was the Massachusetts Eye and Ear. The interview for this position took place with Dr. Harris Mosher, longtime chief of the ENT Department.

"Dr. Curran, I will be happy to consider you, but you must work in our research laboratory for two years. At the end of that time you will be allowed to take the examination for a residency."

That was the quickest brush-off I received since my interview for entering Harvard Medical School. I declined Dr. Mosher's offer and applied to the Brooklyn Eye and Ear Hospital where I was accepted. Their two-year residency paid no salary, but room and board was included. This was the usual compensation for the better residencies.

Duties of a resident in a specialty hospital are similar to service as an interne. Instruction was received in the care of individuals with ear, nose, and throat diseases. During those two years we were given increasing responsibility in the care of patients including all the necessary surgical procedures.

The ten-dollars-a-month compensation I received as an interne at St. Francis Hospital covered most of my expenses, but occasionally I would answer the call for type O blood when my clothes needed refurbishing at the local Salvation Army store.

At the Eye and Ear, I put myself on call at the professional blood agency which was always seeking donors. The fee was $35.00 although $6.00 was first taken out by the agency owners.

One night a call came to give blood to a patient with severe anemia. It was the last time for me as a donor.

The physician taking the blood was considered an expert in direct transfusions which meant that the donor's blood was given directly to the patient. Addressing me during the procedure, he stated, "This patient is also a doctor and I'm sure you wouldn't mind giving an extra 250 cc of blood."

My response was immediate. "I expect to be fully compensated for any blood you remove."

As I watched the dial recording the full amount of blood being withdrawn, I didn't hesitate to remind the physician in charge, "You have removed a total of 750 cc and I expect to be paid for the entire amount."

Several days later the reimbursement check arrived in the mail. It was only for $29.00. When I protested to the agency that the amount of blood taken was 750 cc, their answer was that the transfusion doctor signed for 500 cc and I was entitled only to that amount.

Looking around for other ways to increase my income, I noted that many clinic patients were complaining about spending several hours or more waiting to be seen. Depending on the individual, I agreed to see them in the evening at the clinic rate of 50 cents. This unofficial "fee for service" was pursued without incident, although one patient signaled me from the waiting room area one morning.

"Doctor, I can't see you tonight and my sinuses are bothering me. Can you take care of me now?"

After seating him in the treatment chair and washing out his sinus, he reached into his pocket.

"Shall I pay you today?" he asked.

"Not here, but come with me," I said quietly.

Guiding him into one of the dark rooms that we used to transilluminate the sinuses, I accepted his payment of 50 cents. As he left the clinic I reminded him that my office hours for private consultation were only in the evening.

My after-hours private practice covered the $3.50 round-trip cost of the train which took me from New York to Boston and back. The train left Grand Central at midnight on Saturday and returned to New York early Monday morning. It was a noisy six to seven hour trip, referred to as the Puerto Rican Special, but sleep was usually manageable.

The most popular song at the time was "Deep in the Heart of Texas," which ended with a loud clap, clap, clapping. The majority of the riders didn't know the words, but they all joined in the final noisy applause. This tended to be a rude awakening, but fatigue quickly put me back to slumberland. Best of all, the fare every other weekend, was well within my financial limits.

The Night I was Threatened

"You killed my baby, you killed my baby. Stay there — I'm going to get you."

Hearing these words I was truly frightened not knowing what to expect. Earlier that evening as the covering resident I had been called to see a five-year-old girl who was having a bleeding problem following a tonsillectomy that day.

The surgery had been performed by one of the junior residents, Dr. Torlini, who was not one of our better residents. Whenever a resident signed out for the evening, he was expected to alert the covering house officer of any possible problems relating to his patients. After my review of the history it was obvious that little Wanda had problems during and after surgery primarily related to the control of bleeding.

The bleeding postoperatively was severe enough to require Torlini to bring the patient back to the operating room for resuturing. This complication, distressing to the patient and the doctor, is not common but it is the operating surgeon's responsibility. Torlini failed to remain on duty that night and also failed to alert me that his patient had a continuing bleeding problem.

At the Eye and Ear, about 35-40 operations were performed each day. Any major complications were reviewed by the operating surgeon with the covering resident. Torlini often failed to follow such required procedure and neglected to do so in this case.

Earlier in the day, Torlini had ordered a transfusion which was still connected when I saw the patient. After being notified of the bleeding, a blood count was ordered. This showed a moderate blood loss. Examination of the small black youngster revealed a blood clot in one tonsil area.

I took Wanda back to the operating room, removed the blood clot and resutured the bleeding vessel. I thought that my night's work was done. However, an hour later I received a call from the nurse that Wanda was quite restless. My examination revealed no evidence of bleeding.

Because of her restlessness I ordered a mild sedative, thinking that would solve the problem. But shortly before midnight, I was surprised to get another call. Wanda's restlessness had gotten worse and she was now thrashing about.

After checking her again and not finding any active sign of bleeding, I decided that it would be best to contact the senior attending physician.

"Dr. Lasher, I have a very sick youngster who had a tonsillectomy today and has had intermittent bleeding ever since the surgery. Despite a transfusion and complete control of the hemorrhage, she has become extremely restless. Phenobarbital has not quieted her down. What do you suggest?"

There was complete silence for a moment, then Dr. Lasher said, "Give her a dose of morphine. That should take care of her."

"But Doctor," I replied, "this child only weighs 70 pounds and in her weakened condition I think this would be dangerous for her."

"Young man, do as you are told. I am in charge."

"I definitely do not agree with you, Dr. Lasher," I said. "I'll have the nurse contact you for the order."

I called Wanda's nurse and advised her to telephone Lasher for his order.

It was just one hour later that the call came from the nurse saying she had given the morphine ordered by Lasher and that Wanda's breathing had become very shallow.

"Please come right away," she added nervously.

It only took me a few minutes to get to the little patient's bedside, but her breathing had stopped completely. All efforts at resuscitation failed to bring Wanda back to life. It was now my sad duty to call the the parents. The mother answered the phone.

"Wanda has become quite ill," I said, "and we would like you to come down to the hospital as soon as possible."

The mother appeared at the hospital in the company of her sister about an hour after my call. It took but a few moments to tell the distraught ladies what had happened. I explained the whole problem as gently as I could.

"Wanda had bleeding after her operation," I said, "and in spite of all that was done we were unable to save her life."

As soon as I gave her the news of Wanda's death, the mother collapsed on the marble waiting-room floor. She was a big woman, close to six-feet-tall and weighing at least 200 pounds, and it was with great effort that I was able to get her into a chair where she gradually recovered.

"Call my husband, call my husband," she gasped. "You must call my husband."

After informing the father that his child, Wanda, had died after tonsil surgery his words came thundering through the phone, "You killed my baby! You killed my baby!"

The anger in his voice was disturbing, but the threat that he was "going to get me" was really frightening. After seeing his wife, I was sure that he could match her size and easily carry out his threat of physical violence.

I quickly left the waiting room area and went to my room and changed into street clothes. I called the switchboard operator and signed out to the other resident on service. It was one o'clock in the morning and I wasn't anxious to waken him and try to describe the night's events.

Walking to the subway which was close to the hospital, I took the train to Times Square where I found an all-night movie theater. Seated some distance from me were the usual habitues seeking a warm escape from the cold outside. The film being shown held no interest for me nor for many of the others who occupied seats near by. I felt relatively safe inside despite the closeness of some of the neighbors whose primary concern was the wine bottle they passed around to each other.

At 5 AM I phoned the night nurse supervisor who assured me that the husband had arrived and left with his wife several hours earlier. I returned to the hospital about 5:30 AM and took a short nap for about half an hour. I then arose and showered and got ready to start my day's tour of duty.

It was the end of a night that resulted in tragedy for Wanda and her family. The threat of an anguished parent was something I had never experienced before and it caused me to be understandably fearful.

I have often thought about what could have been done to avoid the tragedy. The resident who performed the surgery insisted that the patient was not bleeding when he last checked her. Some years later a mouth gag was developed that allowed better exposure of an area where Wanda's bleeding probably occurred. It might have saved her life. The morphine injection undoubtedly hastened Wanda's death, but the true cause had to be the surgical procedure and the bleeding that ensued.

I signed out the death certificate: "Cause of Death: Post-tonsillectomy Hemorrhage."

A Patient Who Brought a Smile

She was a pleasant black lady weighing about 175 pounds with a smile that matched her dimensions. Her complaint was an annoying discomfort in the ear that had aroused her from sleep. Finally at 2 AM she called a friend who accompanied her to the Brooklyn Eye and Ear Hospital.

The problem was a large, actively-moving cockroach that had found its way into her ear canal while looking for a warm place to rest. Such an occurrence is not unusual for families who live in poor neighborhoods. Despite good personal housekeeping, the cracks and crevices of their dwellings encourage habitation of many different insects, especially bedbugs and cockroaches.

While examining this moderately apprehensive patient, I reassured her that the problem could be solved in a very short time. Despite my reassurance, I knew there had to be some concern as she was experiencing this bug crawling around inside her ear so I engaged her in some idle conversation.

"Are you married?" I asked while gathering my instruments preparatory to removing the insect.

"Yes," she said, "but I am separated from my husband for five years."

The extraction of this huge insect necessitated small-bite removals, but she continued to answer my questions without hesitation.

"Do you have any children?"

"Yes, I have five lovely angels. The oldest is fifteen and the youngest is two."

Not questioning her lifestyle, but being interested in this charming lady, I then said, "You have a second husband?"

"Oh no," she answered quickly. "I never married again. But whenever I have any troubles I calls him and sometimes when he comes, I weakens."

While saying this, she rolled her eyes and turned and pointed affectionately to a man seated outside the treatment room. He was a little man, barely five-feet-tall and weighing no more than 100 pounds, about half the size of my patient. As she waved to him smiling broadly, he returned her salutation, showing one tooth protruding from his upper jaw, and a tender smile that showed his affection and support.

After noticing these exchanged greetings, I would occasionally glance out to the waiting room while reaching for different instruments. This little man was always in my view, raising his hand in a friendly, encouraging fashion.

In a short while, I was able to complete the removal of the bug. I reassured the patient that she would have no further discomfort. She thanked me effusively while walking back to the waiting room area where she joined her separated spouse.

Arm in arm, they headed toward the exit door where they stopped. She turned and sent me a fond farewell. Still holding her closely as they went out the door, his head was bent towards hers with the same beaming smile that never left his face. I knew in my heart that tonight she would once again weaken.

5

MARRIAGE, MILITARY LIFE, AND ADJUSTING

Military Discipline — AWOL

"Lieutenant, you were absent without leave. Are you aware of the penalty for this violation of duty during wartime? Report to me promptly at 8 o'clock tomorrow morning."

These words were addressed to me on my return from a weekend trip to a resort hotel in Miami.

Prior to my induction into the military, I had paid a farewell visit to Dr. Fitzgerald, a local family physician in Dorchester whom I knew for many years while working at the drugstore. I mentioned that future plans included first, my marriage to Mary Earley, then assignment to army service at Fort Myers.

Dr. Fitzgerald asked, "Where will you be living when you get to Fort Myers?"

"I have no idea," I said, "but I hope there will be living quarters available for both of us close to the base."

This good doctor smiled and said, "That could be a problem. I have a patient who owns an apartment house in that town. Let me see if she might have something available."

Dr. Fitzgerald immediately picked up the phone and spoke with his patient, Mrs. Glover. While holding the phone connection, he turned to me and asked, "Can you and your future wife visit Mrs. Glover at her home in Milton tomorrow afternoon?"

"Yes, we'd be happy to go there," I said.

Milton is a small town near our homes in Dorchester. Mary and I met this lovely woman the next day. We discussed plans for our marriage and the date we expected to arrive at the military post. Mrs. Glover then told us she would be most happy to reserve quarters for us in her complex called the Lincoln Apartments. This building was located in the central part of Fort Myers and easily accessible to the shopping area for our daily needs.

Then came the most unexpected news.

"My husband is recovering from major surgery," she said, "and we

45

won't be able to use our home in Fort Myers for several months. Why don't you live there until we arrive and then you can move into one of the available apartments?"

I was about to ask the monthly rental, but she anticipated my question.

"The rent will be $35.00 a month for the apartment," she said. "You can have our home for the same price."

When we arrived at Fort Myers, Mary and I were completely overwhelmed on seeing our Florida home. The seven-room white colonial house was located on a quiet street, Marilyn Drive, with a spacious yard that bordered the Thomas Edison estate. We were truly in paradise and we immediately sent a note to Mrs. Glover expressing our delight in sharing her beautiful home.

The third weekend of military duty coincided with my birthday on September 21, so we decided to celebrate the occasion by flying to Miami. I checked with the executive officer and told him of my plans.

"No problem," he said flatly.

While waiting to board the plane, an announcement came over the public address system that sounded as if they might be paging me. Mary and I agreed that it must be for someone else with the same or similar sounding name. Nobody knew that we were at the airport except the executive officer and a next-door neighbor, Lieutenant Jensen, to whom we had spoken just a few minutes before we left the house. Ignoring that announcement proved to be a big mistake in judgement.

Our plane took off as scheduled and we had a great weekend in Miami where the weather was exceptionally beautiful. Unfortunately, Mary developed a severe sunburn which took several weeks to heal.

We returned late Sunday night after these joyous few days of rest only to find a note pinned on our front door. It was from our friend, Lieutenant Jensen.

"Please call the Colonel as soon as you return," it said, " no matter how late it is. Urgent."

I was not too concerned after reading the message because I knew that I had followed military protocol in checking my departure with the executive officer. Presumably, I was on safe ground, but I soon learned how terribly wrong I was to make that presumption.

The response from Colonel Fox, after dialing his number, shook me since it was entirely unexpected.

As I stood at attention the following day, the Colonel leaned back in his leather chair with a look of disdain and utter contempt on his face. He reminded me of war movies I had seen depicting a German commander berating a lowly soldier. However, here I was a fellow doctor with the same professional background as the commanding officer. His continuing remarks made me realize that life in the U.S. military is no different than in other countries. Apparently rank has its privileges.

Once again Colonel Fox repeated his message of the previous night, this time with added emphasis.

"Lieutenant, you were absent without leave during wartime. Do you know the penalty for such an offense?"

I was tempted to respond in jest, and ask if he planned on having me shot by a firing squad, but I decided this was no time for frivolous replies. Later, I learned the Colonel had risen from the rank of 1st lieutenant, which was the rank of all newly-commissioned medical officers such as myself. He had decided to make the military service his life career and his status improved rapidly by wartime necessity and not by his medical knowledge or ability.

I remained perfectly silent as he continued, "Your orders were received two days ago for your transfer to Panama City and you were nowhere to be found. This will be recorded in your 201 file."

During my short time in the service I had never heard of such a file, but later I learned that it was basically a record of your military activities. It included reports which could become a stepping stone to a promotion or lead to less desirable transfers if the black marks were significant.

I tried to explain to Colonel Fox that my departure to Miami had been cleared by the executive officer, but this was entirely futile. The *supreme commander* waved his hand at me to indicate that I should remain silent. The Colonel was not finished with me yet.

"In addition," he said, again emphasizing each word as though he was reading a death sentence, "you are guilty of insubordination to a superior officer."

He named Major Fleming as the officer who made the accusation. I again protested that this was not true. The Colonel, at this point, indicated that the interview was finished by handing me a sheet of papers.

"These are your orders and transportation arrangements with the assignment of your next tour of duty at Panama City," he said curtly. "You will leave this post tomorrow morning at exactly 0800 hours."

After leaving the Colonel's office, I thought of the events of the previous three weeks. During that period there was little medical activity to occupy the time of the three dozen or more medical officers in our unit. Most of them, like myself, were commissioned as 1st lieutenants. There were a few of them who had served in the National Guard or Reserves for several years and worked themselves up to the rank of captain or major.

During our required daily attendance at the airfield, nothing very productive ever took place so we spent those hours reading or engaging in discussion periods. Sometimes these bull sessions became heated when we veered off from medical topics to social values, politics, or even worse, a discussion about religion which should have been verboten.

The officer in charge of our group, Major Fleming, was a fat, loud-mouth from Texas. Besides being in charge of our unit, he also thought of himself as having a masterful knowledge of any and all subjects. His response to those of us who questioned his statements was more than most of us could tolerate.

After one of these sessions regarding treatment of ear problems, I made the mistake of contradicting him.

"If you treat an infection that way," I said, "you'll end up with a severe complication, probably mastoiditis."

The others agreed that I was right, but from the look that Fleming gave me, I knew that I should have kept my mouth shut.

The following weekend my name was posted for duty as the Medical Officer of the Day. This required my presence at the airfield where a small clinic had been set up for any emergencies that might need immediate attention. There had been talk of a lottery to pick the medical officers who would be on weekend duty. This suggestion was apparently bypassed at least for the first duty. In retrospect, I realized that Major Fleming had arbitrarily decided on me.

Being on duty at the airfield proved to be pretty dull with little to do medically since the personnel were mostly young recruits who had recently been inducted. The difficulty for me was finding proper transportation to and from the airfield. The bus service was limited to every 90 minutes on weekends instead of every 20 minutes which was in effect during the week.

The medical jeep had been assigned to Major Fleming, but as the O.D. I thought that I might have access to this government property. I approached the Major after getting the assignment for weekend duty.

"Major Fleming," I said, "as the Medical O.D. for the weekend, I will need transportation to and from the airfield. I would like to use the jeep assigned to our unit to fulfill my responsibilities."

"Lieutenant," he answered sharply, "if you don't have your own transportation, you should be living on the post at the B.O.Q. (Bachelor Officers Quarters)."

"Major, my wife and I are living at a house here in town."

"Then in that case I would suggest that you send your wife home," he said arrogantly.

This remark really incensed me. He had pushed me too far.

I turned and practically yelled at him.

"You can kiss my ass."

My response was undoubtedly the reason for Colonel Fox's charge of insubordination and I guess that's what it was. For me, however, it was just one more rude initiation into the disciplines of army life.

After receiving my transfer orders, Mary and I contacted our families in Boston, informing them of our sudden departure for Panama City. We sent a note to Mrs. Glover with sincere thanks for the use of her home. It would be the last home in which we would live together for several years.

The train trip to Panama City was long, hot, and smoky. The steam locomotive emitted ashes and soot through the open-air passenger cars which were probably relics of the first transcontinental railroad. Mary was suffering the agonizing discomfort of her severe Miami beach sunburn. I was burning with the resentment of the events that had taken place during my short indoctrination into life as a member of the armed forces. I realized my actions had precipitated the difficulties but that didn't help.

We arrived at our destination late at night and checked into the only hotel in town. Panama City was a shipbuilding community and it was readily obvious that the hotel didn't qualify as a 4-star establishment. We awakened the next morning to find that our supply of sugar had been invaded by ants.

Flight Surgeon Training

After one night at the only hotel in Panama City, we rented a room from an elderly couple who lived close by the railroad tracks. That was quite a letdown after our delightful accommodations in Fort Myers. Unfortunately, the trains made only two stops at the local station, once at midnight and once at 5 AM, and in both cases the arrival was announced by the loudest whistles possible.

The first week in town we decided to check out the local movie house. We found two seats that seemed comfortable, but halfway through the show the silence was interrupted by the deep gagging and coughing by a patron behind me. His apparent discomfort ended with a monstrous clearing of the throat, ending with an expectoration on the floor next to my aisle seat. A few moments later there was a repeat performance and even in the darkened theater I could see the huge glob of mucus go sailing by me.

I turned and shouted angrily, "Cut that out!"

There was no further expectoration, but when the lights went on at the end of the movie I got a good view of the great grunter and spitter. He was well over six-feet-tall and must have weighed at least 250 pounds. He could have easily disposed of me with one slap of his big, brawny hands. We decided that the only entertainment in town should be off-limits for us.

After visiting the airfield and assessing our living accommodations, Mary and I decided that this was the time to change my status from the medical corps of the air force to that of Flight Surgeon. The application to the School of Aviation Medicine involved considerable paper work going through the various chains of command. There may have been some delay because of the events at Fort Myers and the probable blemish on my 201 file. Undoubtedly, being trained as an ear, nose, and throat specialist would be an added boost to being accepted to flight surgeon training. The need for personnel with advanced instruction and knowledge was especially important as our country became more rapidly involved in the war effort.

The good news arrived about one month after I had sent the information that was required to gain acceptance to being a flight surgeon.

"Your application to flight surgeon training at Randolph Field has been accepted. Report to the School of Aviation Medicine, San Antonio, Texas, on December 15, 1942."

The appointment to flight training necessitated separate travel plans for Mary and me. We agreed that I should go to San Antonio and survey the situation and Mary should return to Boston.

One week after arriving in San Antonio, I found a motel located near the bus which had connections to Randolph Field. When Mary returned to Boston from Panama City, we were forced to be separated for the first time since our marriage three months earlier. This interruption was an established pattern for hundreds of thousands who joined or were inducted into the armed services. There were relatively few who escaped this traumatic situation.

Air flights and Pullman accommodations were practically nonexistent for the average traveler during the war period. Mary's three-day trip to Texas from Boston was accomplished by coach with many train transfers, but we were happy to be together again.

The six-week course at the flight surgeon school was followed by another six weeks at neighboring Kelly Field. It was here that we examined personnel who were undergoing instruction to become members of combat aircraft, including pilots, navigators, and gunners. The training period for air force individuals included spending some time in pressure chambers and it was part of our training to observe the effects of the pressure chamber on their ears, nose, and sinuses. This was pretty routine for me since it involved problems related to my specialty. The entire period at Randolph and Kelly Field went along almost without incident.

Flight Surgeon Yes — Pilot No!

During the program at Kelly Air Base, it was announced that primary flight instruction would be available for the flight surgeons interested in knowing the rudiments of being a pilot. This appealed to me and I accepted this unique opportunity to learn the art of flying as well as experiencing some of the problems.

The instructor was a pleasant individual.

"Have you ever flown a plane before?" he asked.

"No," I answered, "but as a flight surgeon, I'm anxious to know more about what a pilot does."

We climbed into the Piper Cub instruction plane and my attention was directed to the instrument panel which the instructor quickly explained to me. After being seated we became airborne in a matter of minutes and made a pleasant tour of the air field and the surrounding countryside. This was enjoyable and even more so when the pilot said, "You can now take over the controls, but be sure to do as I tell you."

After following his basic instructions, the pilot complimented me.

"You did a good job," he said. "Now I am going to do a few simple maneuvers so keep your seat belt well fastened."

The twists and turns started with what he called lazy eights. These were followed by even more gyrations which my stomach proceeded to imitate exactly. I tapped on the pilot's shoulder and then pointed down toward the ground while holding my other hand over my mouth. He got the message and quickly landed the plane. I then immediately emptied my stomach of its contents.

I staggered away from the plane without further comment to or from the pilot. There was no doubt in my mind that if I looked back I would have seen the instructor convulsed in laughter at another embryo pilot whom he had washed out.

It was a few years later that I met Bob Hoover when he joined the 52nd Fighter Group in Italy. Bob became one of the most sensational pilots in WWII. This is the way he described his reactions when he decided to take up flying as a young man before he joined the air force:

"While learning to fly, I became deathly ill every time I sat down in the plane. I wouldn't actually toss my cookies, but I would become so nauseated that it would almost interfere with my ability to learn. I was determined to stick with it and somehow I overcame my problem."

If I had Bob Hoover's determination to fly I might have stuck with it, but after the initial encounter there was no desire to further my ambition to become a pilot.

During the twelve-week flight-surgeon training, I managed to escape any official reprimand for military discipline infractions, but I did have a close call.

One morning while walking from one building to another at Kelly Field, I met two officers, a tall 2nd lieutenant and a shorter officer. I gave them a wave and a friendly "Hi" while passing by.

The short one stopped immediately and addressed me in the best military tone at his command.

"Lieutenant, is that the way to greet a superior officer?" he said bluntly.

I then noted that he had the insignia of a major on his shoulder pads. Without hesitation I smartly gave him the proper salute and continued on my way. There was no doubt that I still had much to learn about proper army decorum especially with superior officers.

During the time I attended public high school in Boston many years earlier, all students were required to take military drill. Although my grades in all subjects were As and Bs, I never attained much better than a passing C minus in military science. This was an early indication that I was not good army material.

The end of the flight-surgeon training program brought good news and bad news. The names of the successful graduates in the class were posted along with their overseas assignments. That was bad news for some and was probably expected. The good news for me was I had successfully passed my examinations for flight-surgeon status and I was assigned to the E.T.O. (European theater of Operations) where the outlook for a quick victory seemed much better than in the Orient. My orders were issued three days later. I was directed to board a train for New York City.

Mary accompanied me for the two-day trip by coach to New York. As we parted at Penn Station, I waved and cried out "I'll call you tonight." Those were the last words she would hear from me in over two years.

A Seasick Voyage on LST #355

After arriving in New York our group was immediately herded together and placed aboard the LST #355 located at the Brooklyn Navy Yard. The following morning we set sail on a long, unhappy, and somewhat stormy trip that ended in North Africa.

Crammed into a six-by-ten foot triple-bunked stateroom with five other flight surgeons, I was thankful for one thing, that we were all members of the air force and not the navy.

As difficult as it was for the fifty flight surgeons on this craft, it was much worse for the GIs. They were located deep in the hold of the ship next to the heavy equipment for which this vessel was primarily designed. The flat bottom of this Kaiser mass-produced ship caused all the occupants to feel the up and down motion of every wave in the ocean. With the stormy seas that were encountered during the 28-day journey to Africa, there was probably no sea-sickness pill ever made that could give anyone relief on that boat. After a restless night without sleep and with no appetite for food, few of us were inclined to eat breakfast in the morning.

"I'd give a thousand dollars to get off this ship."

This was the early morning greeting that was always received from Brown, one of the flight surgeons who shared our crowded bunk room.

For several days, however, Brownie was the only one who dared to get up and head for the chow line to eat the morning meal. Within minutes of his return he was overtaken by nausea and retching, causing him to deposit his breakfast in the middle of the cabin. This forced the rest of us to leave our quarters immediately for some fresh air. It took three or four of such episodes before Brown agreed to omit the early morning repast.

By the second week at sea, our morning nausea disappeared and we all joined the others for the sunrise meal. When we finally reached the Mediterranean Sea, it seemed like a smooth lake compared to the Atlantic. Once we landed in North Africa, even though we knew we were in a combat zone, it was a blessing after our first, and we hoped our last, naval experience.

General Patton is Reprimanded

"You are nothing but a goddamned coward!"

These words uttered by General George S. Patton, Jr. in a fit of anger, came back to haunt him for some months afterwards.

Our 52nd Fighter Group after several months in Africa, established their next base in Sicily. We were following in the footsteps of the victorious infantry, in this particular case the troops commanded by Patton.

The pilots of our 15th Air Force Group knew that Patton was close by since he had issued an edict that all officers should wear dress caps when off their base. However, the wires in the caps should not be removed.

Most pilots liked the idea of removing these wires because without them the caps could be crushed, thereby supposedly giving them a distinctive appearance. This did not meet with Patton's idea of proper dress. He instructed the military police to give a citation, to be placed on his 201 file, to any officer not observing this military regulation. The pilots resented this infringement on their so-called liberties, but abided by the ruling.

Several of our enlisted men had been admitted to the nearby station hospital because of "yellow jaundice." While not epidemic, some of those affected by this disease were ill enough to be admitted for observation. On this one particular day there was a buzz of excitement with clusters of hospital personnel talking rather angrily.

While visiting one of my patients, I asked, "What's going on around here? It seems that a lot of people are upset about something."

He then went on to explain that General Patton had made rounds earlier that morning with the hospital commanding officer. He approached one soldier sitting in a chair by his bed.

"What's wrong with you, soldier?" he asked curtly.

The frightened private stuttered for a moment and finally answered, "I'm shell-shocked."

General Patton took one of the gloves he was carrying and slapped him across the face, yelling angrily, "You are nothing but a goddamned coward!"

Without further comment Patton continued on his rounds, but the story of the incident spread quickly throughout the hospital and beyond. The members of the hospital staff were enraged by the words and the action of the general, but realized as military personnel there was nothing they could do.

During the next few days, either the media had not learned of the incident or were advised to keep it quiet. Then the whole story broke in the headlines of all the newspapers in the United States requiring the supreme commander, General Eisenhower, to take some action.

Patton was such an excellent general that Eisenhower wrote a formal note to him advising him that he must be more careful in his choice of words and to give a formal apology in front of his troops.

As the war progressed Patton proved his tremendous ability many times over, justifying the faith that Eisenhower had in him. There were many members of the press however, as well as the military, who felt that Patton had been treated too leniently.

A Brave Pilot Loses his Legs to Bad surgery

"For God's sake, Doc, don't send me to a British hospital. Those Limey surgeons will cut off both my legs. They did it to a buddy of mine in England."

While leaning over the injured officer in the rear of the ambulance, I began to wonder if a mistake was being made by transporting our commanding officer to the nearby medical facility staffed by British surgeons. The American hospital in North Africa was 50 miles away in Mateur and was accessible only by winding, unpaved roads in a black-out zone. This was considered too risky in view of the patient's severe wounds.

Several weeks earlier our forces had taken over an airfield in Tunisia. It had been deserted by the Germans whose ground forces had been overwhelmed by the Allies storming through North Africa. On June 19, 1943, the day had been peaceful until the silence was broken by a series of massive explosions followed within seconds by a ringing of the phone in my medical tent.

"Doc, get over here right away. There are bombs going off everywhere at the airfield. All hell is breaking loose."

Within a few minutes our ambulance pulled up at the scene of destruction. It looked as if an air raid had taken place. There were bodies of air force men scattered in the debris and sections of a deserted Nazi plane resting close to the runway. A quick assessment by the other flight surgeons and myself determined that one pilot was dead as well as two other enlisted men. Additionally, there were several dozen more who had injuries that were not life-threatening. The most serious of the injured proved to be the commanding officer of our 52nd fighter group, Colonel Graham West, affectionately referred to as Windy.

The cause of this catastrophic event was later traced to land mines scattered around the airdrome by the Germans before the allied forces arrived. It was also determined that the Nazi plane, a JU-52, had been booby-trapped before being abandoned. This probably was the flash point that ignited the conflagration and set off the explosions all over the airfield. It was never officially determined if inspection of the plane had been done prior to the series of explosions. There was no question, however, that the German objective had been accomplished by the massive destruction that had caused death and injury.

First aid was given to those with minimal injuries. Others were transported to a nearby station hospital which was equipped to treat minor cases of trauma. The most serious wounds were sustained by Windy who had shrapnel wounds of his face with partial loss of his nose, but the worst trauma was the obvious shattering of the bones of both legs with considerable loss of blood.

Tourniquets stopped the bleeding and our supply of plasma helped to improve his circulation although his pulse remained weak and the blood pressure dangerously low. The pain was excruciating and even for a tough pilot like Windy the morphine gave minimal relief.

There was no question that the Colonel's injuries required attention at a facility equipped to treat major wounds. After a quick conference with Alexander, the group surgeon, it was agreed that the American station hospital was not capable of handling major injuries. We were left with no alternatives and we committed ourselves to the British hospital ten miles away. Alexander spoke to their surgeon who agreed to be ready for any operative procedure, so we set out over the winding, unpaved road. Every bump of the uncomfortable journey elicited an uncontrollable groan of pain from Windy. His discomfort greatly increased when I told him that we were heading for the British facility.

I knelt by the Colonel's side and explained why we had to use the British hospital. He at first demanded and then begged, crying out in anguish, "Those Limey bastards will take off both of my legs. They did it to a buddy of mine. Please don't take me there!"

I moved up to the cab of the ambulance where Alexander was seated next to the driver.

"Alex," I said, "the Colonel is vehement about not wanting to go to the British hospital. Do you want to take a chance and try to make the trip to the American hospital in Mateur?"

Alexander turned to me and quickly asked, "How is his condition?"

"Not good," I said. "His pulse is thready and I'm having trouble getting a blood pressure reading. He is definitely weaker and needs whole blood desperately which I'm sure they can supply at the English hospital."

"If the Colonel dies before reaching our own hospital we would be guilty of poor judgement. We can't risk his life."

I agreed. It would be too dangerous to risk the trip to the American hospital.

I moved back to Windy's side and tried to reassure him that he was going to get the best possible attention and it was imperative that speedy action be taken to save his legs and his life.

The Colonel listened to what I said, but immediately followed with his entreaty, "Just make sure you don't let those Limeys take my legs off."

By way of assurance and attempting to allay the Colonel's fears, I said, "Don't worry. We will check the English surgeon's credentials and make sure that he is experienced with cases such as this."

Actually there was no way that we could have immediate access to his capabilities, but I wanted Windy to have some reassurance as he faced the necessary surgical procedure.

The Colonel was not at all convinced. He replied instantly.

"I don't care what you say," he said, quite perturbed. "I wouldn't trust those bastards."

That was his parting angry statement as our ambulance pulled up to the hospital entrance and we delivered him into the hands of the British attendants.

It took but a few minutes for us to meet the surgeon in charge. He examined the Colonel while Alexander and I explained how the injuries had occurred. As soon as Colonel West was transferred to the surgical waiting area, the Britisher turned to us and our hopes for any conservative surgical approach were immediately dashed.

His surly autocratic manner became more repulsive as he minced no words while addressing us.

"We will transfuse the patient and at the propitious moment we will operate and probably amputate."

Our pleas for avoiding possible amputation were completely ignored as the opinion of the Britisher sunk in.

"We will probably amputate." The words reverberated in my head.

I pulled Alexander aside.

"This son of a bitch has definitely decided on amputation unless we can do something to stop him. Try to delay him by any kind of subterfuge and I will attempt to contact the orthopedic surgeon at the American hospital. If he can get here in time we might have a chance to save the Colonel's legs."

A quick review of the map in our files showed an American SAC Headquarters located on the main road to Mateur only three miles away. It was a long shot, but a phone connection could easily be established from SAC to the Presbyterian Hospital Unit in Mateur. My hope was their orthopedic surgeon could be convinced to drive down to the British hospital before any surgery was done and prevent what might be a double amputation.

I outlined my plan to Alexander.

"Tell the Britisher that the American surgeon is related to the Colonel," I said. "Tell him anything but try to convince him that the operation must be delayed."

The whole scenario seemed to fall into place. I made the call from the SAC phone connection to Dr. Thompson, the American surgeon and he agreed to come. I sent Rusty, our ambulance driver, back to the British hospital with the message, "Help is on the way."

While standing alongside the pitch-black road outside the SAC unit, I could not help thinking about the futility of war and its consequences. Almost one hour later the glare of lights came into view. It proved to be the jeep of the orthopedic surgeon, Dr. Thompson. As we headed for the hospital, I quickly explained the concern of the Colonel and the likelihood that the amputation might be taking place.

When I saw the expression on Alexander's face as we entered the hospital, I knew our mission was a failure. Alexander told us that despite his protests and pleas for delay, the surgery was begun shortly after I had taken off for the SAC unit. The British surgeon not only refused to delay the operation, but there was no doubt that he was also determined to perform amputations on both legs.

The three of us walked over to the surgical area where the English surgeon was removing his gown. Dr. Thompson wasted no time in questioning him as to why the operation was done so quickly. The Britisher went on the defensive immediately.

"We had to wait for the propitious moment," he exclaimed, then added, "didn't we?"

While he spoke he winked at his technician who immediately agreed,which I expected. The wink infuriated me and I stood there seething, but there was nothing I could say or do except burn inwardly.

Despite my anger at the English surgeon, the worst revelation was yet to come. Thompson now made a request.

"I want to see both of the amputated legs," he said sternly, "and also place some surgical instruments on the autopsy table."

When the British surgeon hesitated, a confrontation developed temporarily, but the limbs and the instruments were set up as demanded.

The American made his incisions methodically and he held back no punches during his demonstration where he identified each blood vessel and made his comments.

"This left leg had perfect circulation and must have had a pulse, indicating that there was absolutely no need for amputation of any part of the limb."

The English surgeon remained silent. Continuing his dissection, the American surgeon went through the same steps on the right leg.

"These blood vessels are also intact with the possible exception of the ankle, but even that appears to have had good circulation and might have been spared. Certainly from my examination there was no reason for the amputations of these legs."

As the British surgeon blustered again about "operating at the propitious moment," my feeling of revulsion and disgust increased toward this arrogant and incompetent member of the medical profession. The feeling of helplessness was compounded by the realization we had tried everything possible to prevent the crippling of a heroic man.

The words of Windy West came back to me again as they have done so often since that fateful night.

"Don't take me to a British hospital. They'll take both my legs off like they did to a buddy of mine."

Truer words were never spoken.

When Dr. Thompson departed that night, he assured us he would report the entire incident through proper channels.

"My hope," he said, "is that this is one surgeon who will not be allowed to repeat the performance which took away the legs of Colonel West."

In wartime, he noted and we agreed, there was little likelihood that very much could be accomplished.

Alexander and I decided to say nothing about the events that had developed at the British hospital. However, we did inform one of the other flight surgeons of our attempts to prevent the needless surgery. He related the story to the chaplain who was somewhat of a busybody and soon it became common gossip in our fighter group.

I made daily hospital visits to Colonel West and he never once asked me about the decision of the English surgeon to amputate. He talked only about the possibility of flying again. After several weeks of hospitalization in North Africa, Windy was transferred to an American hospital in England.

It was several years later that I learned of Windy West's success in once again flying military aircraft after returning to the U.S.A. He wasn't permitted to return to active duty which he dearly wanted to do. That feat had been accomplished by his hero, Doug Bader, a Canadian fighter who served in the Royal Air Force.

Bader's legs had been removed following combat injuries, but he regained flying status. He also engaged in successful battles with several enemy planes to his credit. Bader was finally shot down and captured by the Germans who could not believe that a double amputee could fly a plane and enter into combat. His successful escape from prison camp ended when he was captured several days later.

Following retirement from the military, Colonel West established his own insurance agency, but died several years later at the age of 44. His death was attributed to bone cancer, but another report indicated he had committed suicide.

Although the actual cause of death appears questionable, nobody can deny the fact that Colonel Graham West loved the military and especially flying. His loss as a combat pilot and leader was something that was unpredictable, but I have often wondered whether we made the right decision that fateful night.

Given the circumstances that prompted our determination to surrender the patient to the care of the surgeon at the British hospital, I have convinced myself that a proper judgement was made. By avoiding the hazardous trip to the American hospital, the Colonel's life was undoubtedly saved. As with any such decision made by a physician in military or civilian life, the tragic consequences of one's reasoning can be disturbing for many years afterwards.

After the war ended, my attempts to contact Dr. Thompson were unsuccessful. This search did bring me in touch with another Dr. Thompson (no relation), who had spent some years at the Walter Reed Hospital as a pathologist during WWII. It was his observation, after examining specimens from service injuries treated in American facilities, that many physicians serving our country were not prepared to treat the combatants efficiently. Dr. Thompson stated that he had examined many specimens that had been improperly removed, usually because the surgeon was not adequately trained to perform the procedures.

Despite a well-trained military force, a democracy such as ours is not fully prepared to adequately face all the medical contingencies in war that are thrust upon the peacetime physicians. We should hope that we will never be involved in any major engagements which will force the mobilization of millions of people, medical or otherwise, to respond to a call to duty on short notice.

Bob Hoover Joins our Group

"Watch me buzz those people on the beach and see what they do."
Equipment had been removed from one of our fighter planes, al-

lowing the P51 to be used as a transport for an occasional passenger with official business. Bob Hoover had agreed to fly me down to the 15th Air Force Headquarters at Bari, Italy, to pick up orders for my return to the the United States. After two years of overseas duty, I was anxious to spend the remaining years of service close to my wife, family, and friends. The trip back from Bari to our home base on the Adriatic coast proved to be somewhat of a hair-raising experience.

While approaching our air field, my exuberant young pilot decided to have some fun. The natives were lounging on the sands enjoying the warmth of the sun. Bob Hoover put the plane into a nose dive and straightened out just before reaching the stretched-out bathers. The plane was low enough to create a hurricane of sand that blew over the frightened beach lovers. As I looked back some of them had risen and were waving their fists at our departing plane. Bob had a broad grin on his face, but I let out a sigh of relief that our journey was ending safely. I was just as scared as the bathers when the plane skimmed barely above the sandy shore.

After Hoover had joined our 4th Squadron fighter Group in North Africa, he was acknowledged and accepted as a superlative pilot and also recognized as especially daring. His rapid advance from flight officer rank (equivalent to sergeant) to advanced officer irritated a few of the less talented pilots who were envious of his accomplishments. Bob Hoover always displayed a great sense of humor and despite his flying prowess, he remained forever young-at-heart.

Shortly after returning to the states, I read that Bob Hoover had been shot down while our fighter group was escorting bombers to a site in Germany. The report stated that he was missing in action. It was many years later that an air show presented in Hartford, Connecticut, featured my hero from the 4th Fighter Squadron. The news article recalled how Bob had become a prisoner of war after escaping uninjured from his disabled plane.

The next day I was able to greet this still very active pilot after he put on a series of acrobatics for the happy spectators. He remembered his days with the 52nd Fighter Group affectionately and he still had his friendly smile.

It was many years later that Bob Hoover once again made the headlines. Chuck Yeager, the first pilot to break the sound barrier, celebrated that historic event by repeating his successful flight on the occasion of its 50th anniversary. This time he accomplished it with a modern F-15 fighter plane. He was joined in this latest dramatic happening by none other than my friend Bob Hoover, who flew a chase plane as he had done before in the original flight.

Return to the U.S.A. — An Unpleasant Welcome

"Soldier, get dressed and go back where you belong or I will stop the train and put you off."

This was an unexpected greeting following my return to the United States some 24 hours earlier.

After two years of overseas duty, orders for my return to the states became effective. Transportation was supplied by a C-47 cargo plane equipped with bucket seats. We departed from Bari, Italy. The overnight flight was interrupted for refueling at Presque Isle, Maine, where we arrived at 3 AM. Arrangements had been made at this stopover for all the passengers to make one short telephone call to their families.

My message to Mary was short and simple.

"I am on American soil and should be in Boston tomorrow night."

Her response was tearful but joyful.

"Welcome home. My prayers are answered."

The plane landed in Washington, D.C. at noon and within a few hours I was at the railroad station checking the schedule to Boston.

I then made one more phone call home.

"All is well. My train is leaving this evening at 6 PM and I should be arriving in South Station by noontime tomorrow. Have the champagne ready."

Every seat was occupied on the train and nearly all were military people. From the chatter I overheard, most of these service men were returning home after several years of overseas duty.

I awoke at 6 AM and the first order of the day was to find a place to clean up and shave. It seemed that everyone had the same idea and the lines to the lavatories were longer than the food queues in the dining area. After walking through the coach cars I came to the Pullman section guarded by a "No Admission" sign. I continued to walk through until I came to a vacant washroom. Closing and locking the door, I stripped down to the waist and started to luxuriate in my new surroundings. The war zone was never like this.

My few moments of glory were suddenly interrupted as the door was unlocked and the blue-jacketed, brass-buttoned figure of the Pullman conductor confronted me. He grabbed my clothes in one swift motion and without any other comment, he shouted, "Soldier, get dressed and go back where you belong."

At first I tried to reason with him.

"There's no room back in the coach lavatories," I said, "and I'll be finished here in a few minutes."

He was not about to give in. His next remark really angered me.

"If you don't leave here immediately, the train will be stopped and I will have you removed forcibly."

My reply was instant.

"Listen, you son of a bitch," I said loudly. "I've just arrived back in the states after spending two years of my life trying to save the hides of bastards like you. Make one move toward me and I'll throw you off first. Now get the hell out of here and leave me alone."

The conductor dropped my clothes on the floor and saying nothing further, left the washroom. It took me ten minutes to finish cleaning up. The conductor never returned.

I retreated to the coach, deposited my shaving kit on the seat and stood in line for breakfast. The Pullman incident was annoying, but quickly forgotten as I later rested back in my seat. I closed my eyes and looked forward to the joy of once again being reunited with my wife, my family, and my friends. There was much for which to be thankful.

Some years later, the April 1992 issue of Harvard Magazine had a New Haven Railroad ad that caught my eye. A picture was captioned, "The kid in upper 4," and the notation beneath it read, "This young man is occupying a berth so he can have adequate rest before embarking on a trip to the Desert War." The readers were furthered cautioned, "Do not be annoyed but grateful for being able to give up your sleep to this soldier who is heading for a potential combat zone."

How times have changed. In 1945 all I wanted was a place to wash and shave after two years in a foreign land.

While I was in North Africa, Sicily, and Italy, I escaped the fatal and the crippling injuries suffered by so many thousands of our military men. When our pilots flew off early in the morning, there was always the concern that some might not return. Almost daily the alert alarm was sounded as enemy aircraft were sighted heading for our airfield. Except for the one mentioned incident, we were spared any casualties at our air bases.

The threatened eviction from the train was unexpected and totally resented as was the reaction of Vietnam veterans when they returned from a war that no one wanted. The media, many celebrities, and some politicians helped to create a sense of animosity against those Vietnam veterans who came back alive, but unfortunately, bore unseen scars. It now appears that the catastrophic war in Vietnam has finally pricked the conscience of the American people and the media. The ad in Harvard Magazine indicated a feeling of compassion for any member of the armed forces who is asked to serve his country.

Military Life in Atlantic City

"Captain and Wife desire Apartment. No pets, No Children."

We placed this ad in the local Atlantic City newspaper after a fruitless search for any reasonably-priced living quarters.

For two weeks following my return from overseas, my wife and I had enjoyed the hospitality of the Ritz Carleton Hotel, courtesy of the armed services. My next assignment for continued duty looked like a real stroke of good fortune.

"You are instructed to report for duty at Convention Hall, in Atlantic City on April 25, at 8 AM."

This appointment would involve examining military personnel, most of whom had been overseas and were being reassigned to other posts. Some were ready for discharge as our infantry and air force were bringing the war in Europe to a close. We now knew where our next post would be and Atlantic City for the summer was an ideal appointment. The problem was finding a place to live.

The duty report was also accompanied by another notice placed in my box at the hotel.

"Your date of departure from the Ritz Carleton is April 20. Please vacate your room by 11 AM on that date."

It was now April 16 and we had four days to find suitable accommodations somewhere in the vicinity of Atlantic City. The city dwellers from the nearby metropolitan areas such as New York and Philadelphia were starting to return to their summer hideaways along the Atlantic shore. They had made their plans some months earlier.

Despite a frantic search for a boarding-house room or an apartment, we were now down to our last day at the Ritz and had been unable to find anything within reason. The ad had been placed in the local paper more out of desperation rather than the expectancy of any response. The rentals offered included abandoned garages, rundown rooming houses, and other such inhabitable places. Anything else was far beyond what we could afford. It looked as though Mary would have to return to Boston and my quarters would be the B.O.Q. (Bachelor Officers' Quarters).

After spending a disappointing day, we returned to our hotel late in the afternoon and found a telephone message in our box.

"In response to your newspaper ad, meet me at 5 PM, corner of California and Pacific. Sam Comly."

It was now 4:45 and we were dog-tired after the long afternoon of fruitless and frustrating searching. With a lot of doubts for any success, we headed immediately for the appointed place. We met Sam, a man well into his seventies, just over five-feet tall, weighing slightly more than 100 pounds, and somewhat slovenly dressed. Neither of us was very much impressed by him, but we decided to see what he had available.

After our introductions, Sam simply said, "My apartment house is at the corner of California and Pacific. Follow me."

He led us at a fast pace to a three-story brick apartment building located a block from the Boardwalk. On reaching the entrance door, Sam stopped and said rather proudly, "This is my building."

We might not have been impressed by Sam's appearance, but after what we had seen the past few days his apartment house looked like a Park Avenue mansion.

Sam then announced, "The apartment is furnished and located on the third floor, but there is no elevator."

We followed Sam up to the second-floor level where he turned and said, "You will have to buy the furniture."

That brought my first question. "How much?"

"The entire four rooms of furnishings, including the refrigerator and stove, is $400."

This seemed reasonable since it meant we would not have to shop around for these necessities.

As we walked into the third-floor apartment, I decided that it was time to find the answer to the $64 question.

Almost holding my breath in anticipation, I asked, "How much is the rent?"

There was no hesitation, but it was a shocker although a pleasant one when Sam answered, "The rent is $36 a month and that is payable in advance."

After seeing so many substandard, unfurnished apartments for $400 and $500 a month, we couldn't believe our ears.

There was no question that we had a real steal, so we thanked Sam somewhat effusively and immediately made out the check for the total of $436.

The next day we signed out of the Ritz Carleton and walked the two blocks to our luxurious apartment. We could not believe our good fortune as we gazed at our new surroundings. Later as we walked down the stairs, we met an infantry captain who had been living in the apartment complex for several months.

After introducing ourselves the captain asked, "How did you ever get the apartment here?"

"You won't believe it," I said, "but Sam answered our ad in the newspaper yesterday."

The captain, Jack Phillips, could only say, "Well I'll be damned."

He then went on to explain what had been happening.

"I have several army buddies who have been on his list for months trying to get an apartment here. Just the other day I told Sam that one of my friends asked about the vacancy on the third floor, but the answer was that it's been taken."

During our conversation with Captain Phillips, we learned that Sam Comly was apparently having some problems with the O.P.A. (Office of Price Administration). that controlled the prices of housing, foods, and other essentials during the war.

Jack Phillips said, "Some families from New York and Philadelphia are now paying 1200 to 1400 dollars a month for a summer rental in this building. Naturally, Sam can make more money from these renters for four months than he gets from the O.P.A. controlled price of $36.00 a month.

The bypassing of the O.P.A. was undetected for several years during the war, but apparently the government agency was now breathing down Sam's neck. The pressure must have hit Sam at just the right time when he saw our ad and decided that he'd better abide by the O.P.A. rules before he got into real trouble.

An Army Snafu and a Happy Ending

On May 8, 1945 the world and certainly the Boardwalk in Atlantic City celebrated the end of the war, officially known as V.E. Day. Anyone in military uniform was glad-handed, kissed by the ladies, and showered with drinks. It was certainly a day to remember, especially for all those individuals who volunteered or were called to serve their country in WWII.

It was several months later that I received some bad news from the personnel section.

"You are hereby notified of assignment to the army station hospital in Spokane, Washington. Your duties will be to head the Department of Ophthalmology. Further orders will follow."

Despite the termination of the war in Europe, there was no indication that the war against Japan was even close to ending. Assignment to a post in the state of Washington seemed to bring me nearer to a combat area in the Pacific.

Mary and I were somewhat in a panic as to what could be done to avoid this unexpected transfer to the west coast. The first step was to notify the air force personnel department that a mistake had been made.

Arrangements were made to see the director at his headquarters in Convention Hall where I presented my case.

"I am not an ophthalmologist," I said to him, "and therefore not qualified to assume the duties and responsibilities of such a specialty. My training is in ear, nose, and throat."

The administrator pulled out the records and pointed to the M.O.S. on my 201 file.

"This identifies you as an eye, ear, nose, and throat specialist," he said in his best military tone, "and this is what we have to abide by."

M.O.S. are the initials for Military Occupation Specialty. The I.D. number on my file indicated that I had been trained as an EENT specialist.

There was no hesitation on my part as I addressed the personnel chief.

"I'm telling you again that I am not trained in eye no matter what the M.O.S. is in my 201 file and therefore I cannot assume the duties of a chief of such a section."

The personnel director was somewhat sympathetic, but reminded me that this information and directive came from headquarters in Washington.

"You may put in a request for a change in your specialty number," he said, "but it may not take effect until after the date set for your tour of duty in Spokane."

Two days later I got hit with more disturbing news. The end of the war in Europe on May 8th had resulted in a point system which was now published. Certain military personnel who had occupational specialties with 100 points or more would be eligible for separation from the armed services if they so desired.

The point system was based on years of service and combat experience and that gave me a total of 110 points. An ENT specialist was eligible if he had a minimum of 100 points. I had the points and the desire and I was ready for discharge. There was only one problem and that was my M.O.S. with the designation as an EENT specialist. The point system required a minimum of 120 points for an eye specialist to qualify for discharge.

I went back to the personnel department once again.

"What can be done to straighten out this mess? I am not qualified to do eye work and my proper M.O.S. makes me eligible to be discharged as of now."

The director of personnel was again sympathetic about my quandary, but he once more pointed out, "These directives come directly from Washington and they move very slowly."

As the days went by, I was confused and somewhat in despair as to what steps could be taken before accepting the army transfer orders to Spokane.

On August 14th, 1945, the prayers of the world and especially the United States were answered when V.J. Day was announced. Shortly after that a new directive was issued stating that all specialty personnel with 100 points or more were eligible for immediate discharge. I was finally off the hook.

After three years of service, there were no regrets about leaving. The war was over and my contribution of two years in the combat zone more than fulfilled my military obligations. More importantly I considered myself indeed fortunate in returning safely and without any physical or psychological scars. There were many within my group who were not as lucky and these young men made the supreme sacrifice.

We sold the furniture in our apartment for $400 to the next tenant who was just as grateful for the trade-off as we had been four months earlier. We cleaned out the apartment of our personal possessions, turned the compass north, and headed towards New England and our future.

6
Private Practice

Class Distinction in Hospital Appointments

The decision to choose a hospital for internship and also private practice was undoubtedly based on some of the prejudices that existed for so many years in medicine. They reached back to the 19th century when the Jewish and Catholic doctors found many doors closed to them.

Starr's book on the "Social Transformation of American Medicine" documents this kind of prejudice that existed in so many of the better hospitals during the late 1800s and up through the early 20th century. During those years, as Starr points out, the elite private hospitals were supported by wealthy patrons. They also sponsored the staff and interne appointments, restricting them to the established families. The Jewish and Catholic physicians were almost totally excluded from consideration in the 19th century.

In Boston, the opening of the City Hospital in 1864 allowed the Catholic and Jewish doctors to obtain staff appointments through their political representatives. Upper class reformers protested the use of this kind of clout in determining admission of patients and doctors to the City Hospital. However, this was something the Brahmins had been doing at the Massachusetts General Hospital since its establishment in 1821.

According to Starr, the MGH did not show outright prejudice to any patients except the blacks. They initially refused to admit Irish patients on the grounds that their presence would deter other people from entering the hospital.

Hospitals, such as the Mass General, gave religious minorities reason for considerable anxiety. Catholics were afraid they might not be given the last rights. Jews were not sure they could get kosher food. Also, both the Jews and the Catholics were worried that attempts might be made to convert them.

When patients of both of these religious groups entered hospitals which were controlled or staffed by members of their own faith, they felt less threatened. However, as late as 1894, such established institutions as Mt. Sinai in New York catered mostly to the aristocratic Jews.

The Russian Jews were of the underprivileged class and they felt uncomfortable and unwanted in such a high-class environment. They preferred the smaller and poorer hospitals run by the Russian Jews.

Jewish and Catholic Physicians in Hartford

I once asked a Jewish friend why he picked Hartford for his professional life. He said the Hartford area was well-known throughout the country for its educational and medical facilities, but especially for its strong Jewish culture.

Many of us are directed or motivated to find our associations on this same ethnic or religious basis. I hadn't done much research or inquired to any great degree about the position of Catholics in Hartford or their acceptance by other religious denominations. I do feel I was indeed most fortunate in deciding to start out my postgraduate medical life in the "Insurance City." The occasional instances of prejudice that did occur during my years of practice were of minor significance and could be found in many sections of the country. More importantly, the welcome mat was out when I completed my tour of duty in WWII and this eased my transition back to civilian life.

In the early years of my practice, I enjoyed good rapport with the physicians attached to the staffs of both Mount Sinai Hospital and Hartford Hospital. In those days there was still a line of cleavage which was recognized and accepted, but in general we all worked together for a common objective, the better care and health of our patients.

Most of the Jewish doctors had appointments at Mt. Sinai where they did the bulk of their work. Some, but not many, were given active staff status at the Hartford Hospital. At that time they realized there was little or no chance of rising above the so-called assistant category and their appointments basically amounted to tokenism. The young Wasps who may have joined the department later were rapidly promoted ahead of them.

Jewish doctors were readily accepted on the St. Francis active staff. The promotions to attending status or heads of departments were sometimes more available to the Catholic physicians since they were in the majority and usually admitted their patients only to St. Francis Hospital.

As the Jewish physician increased his admissions to St. Francis, he ascended the ladder of staff status, becoming associate and chief of the department as readily as the Catholic doctor.

It may seem strange to some, that there should be any difficulty for a physician to admit or care for his own patient in any hospital. How-

ever, the influx of new physicians following WWII created a bed short-
age in the established hospitals. A caste system, or almost a caste system, was developed and became evident as the young doctor came to
town to set up his practice.

The well-established medical facilities, such as the Hartford Hospital, didn't revert to the discrimination that was practiced in the Wasp
institutions of Boston in the 1850s. However, their selection process for
staff appointments was very rigid and made less attractive to the young
Catholic and Jewish physicians who wanted to begin a medical career in
the Hartford area.

The presence of Mt. Sinai Hospital and St. Francis assured Jewish
and Catholic physicians that, if they were properly qualified and wanted
to live in the Hartford area, hospital affiliation was possible at either one
or both of these institutions.

Where to Practice

The doctors whom I knew in Boston were born and brought up within
a few miles from where they decided to practice. Many of my boyhood
acquaintances also tended to remain somewhere in the greater Boston
area. They were truly provincial in every sense of the word.

Dr. Edward Whalen, a mentor during my internship, had encouraged me to choose ear, nose, and throat as a specialty. With military
service behind me, I was anxious to update my knowledge of the latest
advances that had taken place during my three years away from civilian
medical activity. I spent three months in refresher courses in my specialty with advanced instruction taken in Philadelphia, Boston, Baltimore, and New Haven.

As a native of Boston, with friends and family in that city, my first
thought was to seek a future where my roots were established. Before
making that most important decision, I visited Dr. Whalen and asked his
advice.

"I plan on starting my practice in two more months, Dr. Whalen," I
said, "and I'd like to know if you have any suggestions?"

"The place you want to practice," he said, "is the place you want to
live. It's important that you look forward to the years ahead and consider where you want to raise your family. As a doctor practicing a specialty you must have access to a good hospital with equally good staff
physicians with whom you will be associated."

Dr. Whalen never married, but he had a keen insight into the problems of the many doctors he knew and how they resolved their difficul-

ties. As these doctors struggled to maintain a family life and carry on a professional career, he became a silent observer. My admiration for him was based on our limited acquaintance during my interneship and occasional correspondence in the subsequent five years.

"It will probably be more difficult for my wife to adjust to a new environment and find new friends," I said. "My work will keep me occupied, but if she accepts my decision to practice in Hartford, then this will be our future home. Naturally, it's important that I'll be able to admit my patients to St. Francis Hospital."

"If that's your decision," Dr. Whalen nodded, "then I'll be happy to recommend that you receive an appointment to the staff at St. Francis Hospital."

These encouraging words were all I needed to say to my wife, "If you're willing to start a new life in Hartford, we can make plans to move as soon as the baby is born."

Our first child was due in three months, so now I had to find an office and also a place for our small family to live.

Finding an Office

There were no grand developments such as professional buildings when I was ready to start my practice. Office space was limited to large buildings located in the downtown area. These establishments were occupied by lawyers, accountants, architects, insurance agents, as well as doctors. There were no vacancy signs in any of these popular, but not especially attractive places. After much searching, I was able to find an office that was originally a private home converted to professional quarters.

The main office was occupied by an obstetrician. My lease included sharing his waiting room which was quite small. When he was called for a delivery, his patients waited during his absence and that quickly filled the few chairs in the room.

My office space was at the end of the corridor. The obstetrician had his office and three examining rooms off the same corridor.

My small area was large enough for a patient examining chair and doctor's stool as well as a treatment cabinet. A second-hand couch gave me a place to rest at night and for the patient's parent or friend to sit while I examined the patient.

It certainly wasn't Park Avenue, but it gave me an opportunity to get started, while at the same time find a place that we could call home.

Our First Home — The Red-light District

The time for the birth of our first child was fast approaching, but there were no available rentals despite diligently searching through the real estate ads. Buying a home was not possible since we lacked the money for a down payment. Apartments were scarce due to the lack of building activity during the war. The few vacancies that were advertised were well beyond my financial reach.

One of the nurses whom I had known from my days as an interne had heard about my predicament.

"I understand you're looking for a place to live," she said, seeing me at the nurses' station. "A friend of my mother's told her there was a vacancy in her apartment building. Perhaps you might want to see it."

In a few minutes I had the name of the real estate agent whom I contacted immediately. My next stop was Owen Street just a short distance from the hospital and less than a mile from the office space I had just rented.

The four-room apartment was adequate for our needs. It was on the first floor of a three-story building that was relatively clean inside and out. There was no garage, but street parking was allowed. Best of all the price was right, $16 a week. The apartment was partly furnished with a stove, refrigerator, and a few wooden-backed chairs. A visit to the local Salvation Army store would take care of a bed, a crib, and a couple of upholstered lounging chairs. The inside definitely needed a touch-up and Kemtone, the all-purpose paint, took care of that.

Shortly after moving in we discovered that the area had a reputation that was a bit unsavory. It was known as Little Hollywood or the Red-light District. Saturday evenings it lived up to its reputation with a variety of streetwalkers patrolling their territory. The sirens of the police cars on these nights were the only times that the quiet of the neighborhood was disrupted.

I knew that the street was not exactly high-class the day after I moved in. As I got out of my car I heard several loud voices. Two young women living across the street from each other were having a heated argument, Their vocal exchange took place from their third-story apartments. It ended when one of the ladies yelled "Shut up!" The other responded just as vehemently, "Up your ash can!"

There were some wonderful people who lived close by and they helped to make the year we lived in the apartment more enjoyable and acceptable.

There were days that had to be lonely for my wife living in an area with no friends or family. To avoid boredom, Mary would frequently wheel the carriage down the avenue to my office. This also gave our son, Timothy, a chance to enjoy the traffic and the occasional passerby, who would give him a friendly wave. Don't let anyone tell you that being a doctor's wife is a heavenly existence. There were many cobblestones on the road to her husband's success and Mary walked most of them.

Our next move was to a new development of garden-type apartments. After a year in Little Hollywood, this was a giant step forward. The thirty-six months spent in our new apartment proved to be most fortunate and rewarding in those early years. At least a dozen doctors, many associated with St. Francis Hospital, became our neighbors and more importantly, our friends.

During the time we remained there, relationships were established that continued for our lifetime. Our wives played a key role by helping to cement the friendships that had been developed through their husbands' professional associations. The developer and owner of the apartments, Joe Anderson, became a friend and later a neighbor when we built our own home. Joe paid a visit to our apartment area one day. In the midst of the development, he counted eight playpens with children, aged one to three.

As he surveyed the scene, he was moved to comment, "Hasn't anyone around here ever heard of birth control?"

We finally found our Garden of Eden on a one-acre lot where we built a seven-room colonial and raised our three children, Timothy, John, and Elizabeth.

The young physician now beginning practice doesn't endure many of the trials experienced by earlier generations. They are able to marry younger, receive a proper stipend during their hospital training programs, and begin their practice in modern buildings. In addition, they can usually start their lives as physicians in homes that fit their needs and social demands.

These rewards were a long time coming to them, and I for one, feel happy for them.

First House Call — Never Again

"For God's sake, Doctor, help him. He's bleeding to death!"

I had just entered the small home on the outskirts of Hartford and was immediately ushered into the living room where a man, in his late 40s, was stretched out on a sofa. Blood was streaming from his nose and the dried material was caked on his face and arms. His bathrobe, pajamas, and the carpeting beneath him were matted with blood-stained vomitus. Surrounding the patient were three women and two men, all relatives of the family. One of the women, his wife, glared at me as she demanded that something should be done and immediately.

For me, it all started at 2:30 AM, when a call came from the family doctor.

"One of my patients," he said, "is having a severe nosebleed. He lives in Elmwood and I told the family that you would take care of it right away."

The doctor gave me the name of the patient and the address and quickly hung up, leaving me to find the house in the small suburb of West Hartford, Connecticut.

The short time I had been in practice gave me no opportunity to know the geography of the towns surrounding Hartford. During my one-year interneship six years earlier the only transportation I used was the local bus line.

Fortunately, a local policeman seated in his patrol car alongside of the road noticed my car as I slowly drove down the unfamiliar streets. Recognizing the M.D. on my license plate, he pulled up to my car.

"What's the matter, Doc?" he said. "You look lost. Maybe I can help."

In a matter of a few minutes, he guided me to the proper street and residence where I faced the patient who was obviously in need of help. He was a huge man, well over six-feet tall, and possessed a gigantic head, large sinewy arms, and enormous hands.

There was no difficulty in recognizing him as an acromegalic, an individual who was suffering from an overactive pituitary. The victims of this disease are frequently seen in the sideshows at the circus. Their musculature gives them an opportunity to display their great strength when they are seen on the stage. However, their condition makes them subject to a marked elevation of blood pressure which can cause severe nosebleeds and often brain hemorrhage.

The three women stood over me almost menacingly as I unpacked my bag of medical instruments. Their presence disturbed me, prompting me to say, "You must leave this room immediately while I take care of this very sick man. Go into the kitchen or the bedroom, but don't come out until I call you."

They left muttering in Italian, which I recognized as their native language, but fortunately did not comprehend what they were saying. They were noticeably angry at being told to leave the room and probably cursing me as they walked out, figuring that I wouldn't understand the language they alone understood.

I then turned to the two husky men, who identified themselves as brothers of the patient.

"Angelo," I said to the patient. "Listen carefully and do what I say. I want your brothers to bring you up up to a sitting position on the sofa. I don't want you to slide down."

As the patient was brought upright, he immediately vomited bright red blood clots that further drenched his robe and the blankets that surrounded him. The floor was already covered with a considerable amount of dried blood and vomitus that had erupted for sometime before I arrived.

The brothers now looked at me and watched the blood that was pouring from the patient's nose and mouth. They were convinced that if Angelo was forced to lie down as they had him before, there would be no bleeding. It was time to explain to them that the blood they did not see was being swallowed and filling the stomach when he was forced to lie flat and that produced the vomiting.

The next part was going to be the most difficult for the patient, the brothers, and the doctor. It would be necessary to put a gauze plug into the back of the nose to control the bleeding.

I gave the instructions to the brothers once again.

"You must hold Angelo in a sitting position while I stop the blood. Don't let him move if you want me to save his life."

Showing them a twelve-inch rubber catheter, I now attempted to explain what I was going to do.

"I will put this catheter into his nose until it comes out of the back of his throat. Next I will tie this gauze roll to the end of the catheter. When I pull the catheter back out of the nose, the gauze packing will be in place directly on the bleeding point in the posterior nasopharynx, which is the back of the nose, and that will stop the bleeding. What I'm going to do is going to be very uncomfortable for Angelo, but there is no other way to help him."

Both brothers looked at me somewhat incredulously, but said nothing. It made me wonder if either or both would collapse before I was able to complete the pack insertion.

Next I explained to Angelo what the steps would be and how important it was to have his full cooperation. He showed the same reaction as his brothers, a look of fear and apprehension because of his natural concern about the continuous bleeding.

With the headlight adjusted properly, I carefully inserted the rubber catheter into Angelo's nose and grasped it as the end protruded into the back of his throat. I then tied a prepared rolled-up gauze packing to the end of the catheter and gently pulled the rubber tubing back out of his nose, watching the gauze packing slide into the back of the throat. First placing a mouth gag between the patient's jaws to prevent him from biting down, I inserted my finger into his mouth and guided the packing into its proper position in the posterior nasopharynx where the bleeding point was located. The mouth gag placed between Angelo's huge jaws definitely saved my index finger from a serious bite as his jaws came down hard. A non-surgical amputation could easily occur without such a precaution as I made the final adjustment of the gauze packing.

The operation was a success, but caused the patient to scream with discomfort as the procedure was being done. The women immediately came out of the kitchen in an attempt to comfort Angelo. At the same time their looks and their comments in Italian indicated I had inflicted unnecessary pain on the patient. After assuring them that the nosebleed was under control, I advised them that hospitalization was required for blood counts, transfusion if necessary, and observation.

The ambulance was called and after cleaning my instruments and wiping the blood off my hands and face, I left for the hospital. I checked Angelo once again when he arrived in the emergency room and wrote the admission orders. I spoke to Angelo's family who were gathered there. They no longer seemed menacing, but appeared more apprecia-tive of my successful efforts to stop Angelo's frightening hemorrhage.

It was close to 5 AM before I returned to my office apartment. Re-viewing the night's events, I had to admit that my first house call was not very satisfying for several reasons. A severe nosebleed can be a trau-matic experience for the patient and the physician and the family.

The patient and his family are naturally terrified when they see the constant hemorrhage and they look for a quick and painless response from the doctor.

Most patients will survive the loss of blood after emergency mea-sures are administered in the hospital where proper and complete care can be given. Bleeding from a large blood vessel in the neck or extremi-ties which often occurs in accidents requires immediate attention. How-ever, the blood flow from the nose will usually diminish as the blood pressure drops. This allows adequate time for the patient to be hospital-ized for transfusion and control of the bleeding under ideal circumstances. The first house call taught me a valuable lesson. After that experience, future patients with similar problems were advised to go immediately to the hospital where emergency measures and competent assistance would be available for me so that I could do my job properly.

The days of kitchen surgery, however dramatic, have long since passed.

Jack the Ripper Strikes

"Doctor, I had my tonsils taken out by Dr. Priory and my friends can hardly understand me when I talk. What is wrong?"

The patient with the complaint had been examined by me some six weeks earlier. She had a history of severe recurrent sore throats for almost one year. During that time she had been seen by the health clinic nurse and doctor at one of the local insurance companies where she worked as a file clerk. The company physician suggested consultation with a throat specialist for a possible tonsillectomy.

The patient, Marilyn, had markedly enlarged tonsils when I first saw her with some swelling of the glands in her neck, a definite indication of severe infections in the past. In view of the examination and the history, I advised tonsillectomy. The accepted routine in my early years of practice was to have the preoperative physical performed by the family doctor.

"Marilyn, do you have a family doctor?" I asked. "You must have a physical examination before the surgery."

"No," she answered, "but my friends will know someone they can recommend."

"Good. As soon as you have the physical, bring in the doctor's form and you will be booked for the operation."

Unknowingly, I had stepped into one of the major problems encountered by the younger surgeons after returning from service. It was the common practice of some family physicians to assist or perform surgery. They often assisted the general surgeon on the case they had referred for major surgery. This would usually allow the assisting doctor to charge a fee for his services. It was a cozy arrangement that kept the surgeon happy as well as the patient who would be seen each day by the family physician. Not all the surgeons entered into such dealings, but it was tolerated although frowned upon by those who did not participate in this shady system. Surgical nurses were usually more adept at passing the instruments than the family doctor who occasionally filled in as an assistant.

Dr. Priory not only was allowed to help the surgeon, but he also had privileges in tonsil surgery and obstetrics. The latter arrangement permitted him to deliver babies without any assistance from the staff obstetrician. He was expected to call in the specialist, if needed. He ran into difficulties frequently causing complications that prolonged the patient's hospitalization.

If the mother happened to have a large baby and there was a problem in delivering the child, Dr. Priory was inclined to use a little more force. This often ended up with a tear which required repair by an obstetrician at a later date. This family doctor had earned his title of "Jack the Ripper" from some of the obstetricians who complained, but without success, that he shouldn't be allowed to deliver babies.

After starting my practice of ear, nose, and throat, Dr Jack was still doing obstetrics as well as tonsil surgery. He maintained a good liaison with some obstetricians, since he was a source of referral for gynecological cases such as tears in the birth canal which he himself caused.

It was two weeks after first examining Marilyn and recommending tonsillectomy that her name appeared on the operating-room schedule. She was listed for the tonsil procedure that I had recommended, but the surgery was to be done by Dr. Priory. I was annoyed and angry by what had happened, realizing that the case had been literally stolen from me. However, the patient has the right to choose the physician of his or her choice, no matter what the treatment, medical or surgical.

Now Marilyn was in my office again, six weeks after she had her tonsillectomy by Dr. Priory. Before I looked into Marilyn's throat, I said, "Why did you have Dr. Priory take out your tonsils? You had already agreed to have me do the surgery."

"When I saw him for the physical exam, he said that he did lots of tonsils. He also told me that you were just a young doctor without his experience. That's when I decided that it might be better if he did the operation. I know I made a terrible mistake, Doctor, but do you think you can help me?"

"Let me take a look inside your throat first, Marilyn," I said gently. "By the way, when you drink liquids, do they come out of your nose?"

"Yes, Doctor, they do. And when I saw Dr. Priory last week, he told me that my voice and the liquids coming out of my nose would clear up shortly. It's been over a month since my operation and I still have the same trouble."

When I looked into the back of Marilyn's throat, there was a large gaping hole above where the tonsil had been on the left side. The soft palate was almost completely gone on that side. The soft palate is like a "curtain" or flap of tissue that hangs over the back of the throat. It has several purposes. When we swallow the "curtain" closes down and prevents liquids from going into the back of the nose and out the front.

When we talk the "curtain" also closes and that prevents air from our lungs rising back into the nose and producing a nasal speech.

Some children are born with a condition called cleft palate in which the soft palate fails to develop properly. These children have a nasal speech and swallowing problems until corrective surgery is performed. Any injury to the soft palate may cause the same symptoms.

Dr. Priory had taken a short course in New York where the participants, usually family doctors, were instructed in the use of the Sluder for removal of tonsils. This technique required pushing the tonsil into the loop of the instrument which was clamped around the diseased lymphoid tissue. The surgeon then used his finger to separate the tonsil from its bed.

Any patient with a long history of throat infections develops considerable scar tissue which requires removal with a knife or scissors. Dr. Jack, apparently unable to dissect the tonsil out with his finger, must have given the Sluder instrument a strong pull upward, ripping off the soft palate along with the tonsil.

On examining Marilyn's throat and seeing the large hole on the left side of the soft palate, I became angry and frustrated by this kind of careless surgery. But I was anxious to alleviate her problem.

"Marilyn, I believe that we can correct your problem. Come back to the office in one week and I'll tell you what has to be done."

Some weeks earlier, Dr. Kazanjian, a world-renowned plastic surgeon presented a talk at the Massachusetts Eye and Ear. He described his experiences in treating shrapnel wounds of the head and neck, especially those with damage to the soft palate. It seemed quite possible that his method of repair could be utilized in closing the gaping hole in Marilyn's throat.

The notes from Kazanjian's lecture and a review of his book on soft palate repair convinced me that this patient could be helped. There was no plastic surgeon on our staff at this time and Marilyn's insurance would not begin to pay for hospitalization and treatment in Boston.

When she returned a week later, I explained what had to be done, but was careful not to offer any iron-clad promises. Based on my knowledge of the anatomy in the throat and my surgical experience in the army, however, I felt confident of success.

At the time of surgery ten days later, I carefully undermined a large flap of tissue from the inside of Marilyn's left cheek. I then brought one end of this elevated flap over to the opening left by the loss of the soft palate and sutured it to the remaining torn edge of the palate. The other end of the cheek flap was left attached to maintain a good blood supply.

I inserted a nasal feeding tube which remained there for ten days as the tissues healed. Marilyn was then discharged.

In two months Marilyn's throat was completely healed. Her voice was almost normal and the liquids she swallowed no longer came back through her nose. Such a case never came to my attention again, but in later years qualified plastic surgeons came on our staff. They certainly are the proper specialists for treating those cases and other problems beyond my training and competence. However, as new techniques were developed in the field of ear, nose, and throat for the control of previously unmanageable problems, I joined the parade of those seeking new horizons.

It was shortly after Marilyn's successful recovery that I met Dr. Priory in the hospital. Directing him into a quiet corner, I held back no punches while expressing my thoughts.

"You deliberately stole that patient who came to you for a preop physical. You actually butchered her throat with your surgery and I was fortunate to obtain a good repair. What do you have to say?"

Priory sputtered and then became almost defiant in defending his surgery.

"I have taken out many tonsils," he said, "and never had a problem before."

"You have been doing most of your tonsillectomies while the other throat doctors were in the service. Who has been around to check your work? You can avoid more difficulties by not doing tonsil and adenoid surgery in the future."

As Priory made a hasty retreat, I made no mention of the possibility of malpractice, since in those days such actions occurred mostly in the larger metropolitan areas and were uncommon even there.

Jack the Ripper Strikes Again

It was some weeks after Marilyn's misfortune that another case of Dr. Jack's surgical misadventures occurred. A call came from Dr. Sam, the ENT physician covering one evening. He had been asked to see a five-year-old patient who had been bleeding following tonsil surgery by Dr. Jack earlier that day. Dr. Sam stood by as I examined little Jane.

"I looked in her throat in the operating room twice this afternoon," he said, "but I didn't see any bleeding. She was sent back to her room, but each time she vomited a basin full of blood about an hour later, so I know she's bleeding. What do you think, Tim?"

Dr. Sam talked to me as the patient was being put to sleep and I explained what may have happened and what should be done.

"The best way to see the throat is with this relatively new mouth gag. It allows you to see areas which might not otherwise be visible."

After inserting the mouth gag, I pointed to a large blood clot well below where the tonsil had been removed.

"You can now see the blood oozing from that clot," I said, "and flowing down into the stomach."

It took just a few seconds to remove the blood clot and reveal a pumping vessel that was easily clamped and tied. Dr. Sam readily admitted that his old-fashioned mouth gag couldn't possibly expose the bleeding point that had developed.

Little Jane required one more unit of blood to replace what had been lost and was discharged from the hospital three days later.

The use of the Sluder tonsil instrument had produced a tear downward in this child's throat. The bleeding occurred below the tonsil area and thus was difficult to visualize. It produced severe blood loss which became life-threatening despite replacement by transfusions. The pulling of the Sluder upward during Marilyn's tonsillectomy caused loss of palatal tissue. In the child's case the tearing of the membranes below the tonsil opened up several large blood vessels which were potentially dangerous, but were easily found and sutured.

After Jane was discharged from the hospital, I called Dr. Priory and angrily told him in no uncertain words, "Enough is enough. You have grossly mishandled two cases that have come to my attention. I'm going to request the surgical executive committee to withdraw your privileges for tonsil surgery."

There was silence at the other end of the phone for a few moments. Dr. Priory then answered, "I've been doing these operations for many years and no new doctor like you is going to stop me."

Jack the Ripper Strikes Out

Dr. Priory hung up after his fiery statement. I decided to take the bull by the horns and contact the surgical executive committee of the staff by formal letter. Two weeks later in response to my complaint the committee chairman asked me to attend their monthly meeting and discuss my suggestions.

It was a real eye-opener as to how some doctors, especially those from the old school, think. Some of them resented the entry of younger doctors coming onto the staff and bringing new ideas.

I gave my presentation.

"No qualified physician," I said, "should be deprived of caring for his patients, whether it is a surgical problem or a medical disease. However, Dr. Priory has demonstrated a lack of skill in performing tonsillectomies, no matter how many he may have done in the past."

Several questions were addressed to me by the committee members and I answered them to their apparent satisfaction. However, one question from Dr. George, a general surgeon, really annoyed me.

"Dr. Curran, if Dr. Priory is not doing the operation properly, then you should teach him the right way."

I quickly responded, "Dr. George, it took me two years to learn when and how to do this procedure. If you really feel that way about surgery, why don't you show him how to take out an appendix or fix a hernia?"

My comments brought about a few agitated remarks from the surgeon, but the rest of the committee showed general agreement with my presentation.

One week later I was notified that Dr. Jack's privileges for tonsil surgery had been terminated. The following month the members of the obstetrical staff, emboldened by my success, requested that he should not be allowed to deliver babies. For several years this was a permission that had also been tolerated despite the fact that his ineptness had caused numerous complications. The executive committee agreed with the obstetricians' recommendation.

For several months after Dr. Jack's privileges were curtailed, there were a few less requests for ENT consultations from some of the family physicians. The word had been passed around that I was unfairly preventing one of their members from performing surgery. The vast majority of family doctors, however, didn't do any surgery and their referrals continued without interruption.

A Bleeding Tonsil and a Father's Power

"Your last tonsil is bleeding. You better get up here fast and check him out."

It was the OR supervisor calling about an hour after finishing my last case. The patient was a nineteen-year-old young man, Robert St. Clair and after examining him in the recovery room I found a large blood clot in the left tonsil fossa. Such a thing happens occasionally despite careful suturing of all bleeders at the time of surgery.

I explained this to the patient.

"Robert, I'll have to take you back to the operating room and stop the bleeding. You should be able to go home tomorrow as scheduled."

"Before you take me back to surgery, Doctor, would you please call my father? He has the power to stop bleeding."

I was anxious to take care of the problem immediately, but understanding the young man's concern and faith in his father's ability, I asked, "How do you know your father has this power?"

"He received it from his father and it has been passed on for many generations. My sister had her tonsils removed about fifteen years ago when we lived in New Hampshire. She was five years old and the doctor couldn't stop the bleeding. After two weeks my father used his power and the bleeding stopped."

"Robert, I am sure your father has the power, but hospital rules only allow doctors in the operating room. It's necessary for me to do the suturing immediately."

The supervisor walked into the recovery room.

"What are you planning to do with this patient?" she said.

Keeping a straight face I said, "The patient says his father has the power to stop bleeding so I thought we should bring him in for consultation."

Nora Walsh, who usually kept control of herself, let out a bellow that must have been heard in the entire operating area.

"Will you get your ass into the scrub room and stop horsing around. You're holding up the OR schedule."

After controlling the bleeding, I contacted Robert's mother and explained why suturing had to be done. I asked her about her husband's power.

"My daughter bled so much that we thought she was going to die. The doctor agreed to have my husband use his power and the bleeding stopped right away. He saved her life, that's what he did."

"Doctors Gouge the Public"

"Doctors make a million dollars a year. They gouge the public."

These words were uttered by an insurance executive whose income, he admitted, averaged close to one million dollars yearly. I had heard this statement before, expressed in different ways and words by several other acquaintances.

These individuals, in various segments of business and other professions, were highly successful in their chosen fields and were well rewarded. They admired their friends and associates who were also in the upper income level. However, this admiration didn't extend to physicians who attained success only by total dedication, sacrificing sleeping hours and vacation time to assure personal care to their patients.

Most physicians have worked long hours and spent additional days and weeks in improving their skills and knowledge by further training to adapt to the changes in medical care. The number of doctors who reach the million-dollar-income level are few and far between and are often entrepreneurs or sometimes charlatans. Overall, they don't represent the physicians that I have known.

I've thought back over the years, not only of my own medical life, but also of the physicians with whom I was associated. These doctors had the same philosophy that I tried to embrace and they followed their ideals to the letter. The primary concern of most physicians has always been the health of the patient. Fees were never involved in our treatment when we made decisions about the care of the individual who sought our advice.

I realize that there are physicians who are motivated more by the dollar sign than the Hippocratic Oath. They existed in the past and they exist today. In more recent years, especially, I'm shocked at the billing charges of some doctors. Although they represent a small minority, I can readily understand why universal health coverage has such widespread appeal.

Despite a desire to give back as much as possible to the community, there was some disenchantment after several years in practice. I had become a participating physician in Blue Cross and Blue Shield as soon as it was established in Connecticut. The fee schedule was much lower than many ENT physicians found compatible with the rising costs of practice and the increased expenses of maintaining their households. Many doctors, including most of my ENT colleagues, decided that failure of BC/BS to raise their fees left them no alternative. The majority of these doctors refused to participate and proceeded to charge fees that were higher than the BC/BS allowance, but still fair to the patients for the specific procedures performed. The established schedules had been set low to allow low-income participants to have private care without additional charge. Under those guidelines, I decided to remain a participating physician and a member of the organization. I truly believed that there was a place for such an insurance plan.

Soon it became evident that many individuals who declared their income below the acceptable level for service benefits were obviously lying. The established income level had been set at $5,000 which at that time appeared reasonable. Although it was evident that some families were well above the so-called maximum, I continued to accept the statement of the members that they qualified.

About one year following the mass exodus from BC/BS by the ENT physicians, I decided to join them. My office expenses, including malpractice and other insurance costs, were sky-rocketing as well as the personal costs of maintaining a home with three children. Most disturbing were the patients whose living accommodations were far above what I could afford and yet they had the brashness to seek service-benefits protection with their BC/BS insurance program.

With some reluctance, I sent in my resignation from a group that failed to recognize that the cost of living affected doctors also.

"Save my Child's Eyesight, No Matter What the Cost"

I received an urgent call late one evening to examine a youngster who had developed a sudden swelling around his eye. The family had called Dr. Mancall, an eye specialist, who recognized that the problem was the ethmoid sinus.

I met Dr. Mancall in the emergency room where he explained the problem.

"When I saw little Tommy a short while ago I ordered sinus x-rays immediately. Although the eye was protruding, my examination was otherwise essentially negative and I knew that we had a serious sinus problem on our hands. What do you think, Tim?"

I examined the five-year-old child, checking the nasal passages and the eye. There was no question as to the diagnosis.

"The redness and the swelling around the eye," I said, "is typical of ethmoiditis and the x-rays confirm your original impression. If we rely on antibiotics, the pressure of the pus may cause irreversible damage to the eye before the drugs take effect. Surgery is the quickest and surest way to avoid a blind eye."

We now talked to the parents and while showing them the films we explained the seriousness of the problem.

"These cloudy areas are the ethmoid sinus cells. They surround the eyeball with pus which can break through and may cause loss of vision, even blindness. If I operate tonight, the sinuses can be drained and help clear up the infection. Any delay certainly is not advisable."

The father, an executive with one of the major manufacturing companies in Hartford, became insistent as he demanded, "Tommy must have the best of attention and I want you to bring in the best specialists from Boston or New York, if necessary."

I now felt the parent was becoming unreasonable.

"You may call any specialist you wish," I said, "and I will bow out of the case. The choice is yours."

The father immediately became apologetic.

"Save my child's eyesight, no matter what the cost. Do what you think best, Doctor. I have complete faith in your judgement."

The operation presented no problems. The patient recovered with normal vision and was discharged from the hospital a few days later. The family was effusive in their appreciation.

Nobody could have been more grateful.

When the child returned for a final checkup at my office, the mother presented several insurance forms of companies that covered the surgery.

About three months later my secretary approached me with a problem.

"What should be done about the Johnson boy's bill? I have contacted the insurance companies and asked if the billings were in order and they assured me that the policyholder had been reimbursed in full."

I reviewed the chart and the account and noted that the total payments to the parents more than compensated my billing of $150 which covered my surgery and all visits.

Several months later my bookkeeper suggested that the account should be referred to a collection agency. We rarely had occasion to do something like this since more than 90% of our patients responded to our billings. The threat of such action in this case brought immediate payment from these demanding and delinquent parents.

Over the years, in my experience, the vast majority of patients, especially those in the middle class or lower income group do pay their bills. Far too often the problem was with the family that lived in the big house, drove the luxury car, and had membership in the exclusive clubs. They demanded the most, and far too often they were listed among the worst offenders.

"Hell Doc, You're a Sucker"

I received a call one afternoon to see a youngster at the McCook Hospital. This hospital was supported by the City of Hartford and was primarily for the indigent. Many doctors like myself gave freely of their time on a regular basis for these patients.

Service at McCook required spending one morning a week, seeing patients in the clinic and operating on patients who required elective or emergency surgery. My commitment was for six months each year. It was no big sacrifice, although it meant giving time that could be occupied in taking care of private patients or spending the extra hours with my family.

On this one occasion the young boy I saw was suffering from severe croup which required an emergency tracheotomy The rest of my office appointments were canceled while I performed the surgery. The patient recovered successfully and I followed him in the hospital until his discharge. Later I saw him in the outpatient clinic until his wound was healed. I never inquired into the financial status of the family since I presumed that the hospital administration screened all admissions as to eligibility for free care.

Some months later the father of the young boy came to the office for an ear problem. On the financial history taken by my secretary, she had asked him his occupation.

He replied, "I'm a builder."

While readying my instruments for the examination, I asked, "How is the sale of houses these days?"

"Very good," he answered. "In fact I've sold two this past week and I'm just starting another one."

It was then I noticed on the chart that he was the father of the youngster on whom I had done a tracheotomy several months earlier.

"Tell me," I said, "how did you have your son Robert admitted for an emergency operation at McCook Hospital instead of having him seen at St. Francis or the Hartford Hospital as a private patient.?"

His reply was somewhat of a shocker.

"Our pediatrician recommended you for the surgery," he said, "but I was told that you were also on the staff at McCook Hospital. I asked myself why should I go to the St. Francis Hospital and pay all those fees when I could have it done for nothing."

At this point I gave him an angry response.

"I give time without charge to poor people who cannot get proper care unless I offer my services completely free."

"You mean," he said surprised, "you don't get paid by the city?"

Almost mimicking his words, I said, "No, I don't get paid by the city."

His response really floored me.

"Hell Doc," he said sarcastically, "you're a sucker."

Over the years, along with many of my colleagues, I guess, at times I've been a "sucker." There have been occasional moments of chagrin and disappointment in some people who have taken advantage of a possible free ride. However, they are definitely in the minority.

I've never regretted the steps taken in trying to assure my patients, no matter what their economic status, of the best care that could be offered. There aren't too many professions or businesses where one is in a position to do so much for so many and have sincere gratitude from those who received your care.

It is most unfortunate that there is no true appreciation by some people of the free services rendered by physicians in the past and even in the present day. Most doctors enjoy their work in medicine and aren't looking for plaudits. Like myself, they just resent the unfairness of the critical comments that they sometimes receive.

A Mother not Impressed by the Nuns

"Dr. Curran, I want to cancel arrangements for my daughter's operation."

Canceling surgery is not too uncommon, but this mother's explanation really floored me. I received this telephone call after I'd been in practice for only a few years. The patient was a referral from one of the pediatricians.

Mary Ann, a four-year-old child, had multiple attacks of tonsillitis with high fever. Despite the use of antibiotics, she became subject to increasingly frequent sore throats. She also developed severe mouth breathing causing her to have restless nights and poor sleeping habits. When the referral was received, I knew that she must have been experiencing a lot of problems because her pediatrician was opposed to tonsil surgery except in extreme cases.

After my examination and review of the history with the mother, I told her that surgery was indicated. Sensing that the parent was not too keen about the operation, despite my explanation, I called the pediatrician in the presence of the mother. Agreement was reached to have the surgery performed and arrangements were made for the child's admission two weeks later.

The day for admission finally came with surgery scheduled for the following morning. The mother called to say that she wanted to cancel the operation. I was ready to accept her decision without any question, but she immediately went on to explain the reason, going into great detail as I patiently listened.

"My husband and I have been married for ten years," she said. "We waited a long time before Mary Ann was born. We have never left her alone during these past four years except on one occasion. We hired a sitter and went out to a restaurant to celebrate our wedding anniversary.

Just as dinner was being served I decided to call the sitter to see how Mary Ann was doing. When she told me that our baby was crying, we left the table without eating our meal and we have never left her alone since that time."

I thought that would end the conversation, but she had more to say.

"We know she has a lot of problems with her throat and that surgery should be done, but then my husband and I talked about how she would react after the operation. These nuns, all dressed in black, would look just like witches to her and she would be scared out of her mind."

The nuns, of course, didn't dress in black, but were gowned in white when working on the wards. On occasion, if the mother was concerned about leaving the child alone because of the patient's or parent's apprehension, I would suggest that the mother might wish to stay with the youngster during the hospitalization.

Usually this meant that the mother had to sit in a chair by the bedside for the two-night stay. In this instance I didn't make this suggestion. It just didn't seem like a practical solution.

I thanked the mother for calling me and I notified the pediatrician of the cancellation and the reason given. I never learned whether the mother sought consultation with another ENT physician for her daughter's surgery.

With all the concerns that overwhelmed the mother, it would place the doctor under a cloud of apprehension. Even the smallest complication would have created a lot of aggravation for any surgeon. In the minds of the parents there might have been considerable second-guessing, especially if they had made the decision to have their child admitted to a Catholic hospital. Any nightmares or psychological problems of their child would undoubtedly be related to the witch-like (black habit) or ghostly appearance (white gown) of the nuns.

There were no similar incidents during my many years of practice. The nuns continued to give the patients, the nurses, and the doctors the solid support that was so necessary in maintaining their high standards.

Confrontation with the Law

Often times I've wondered about the choice of ear, nose, and throat as my specialty. It was the call to see the patient with a severe posterior nose bleed that all too frequently put doubts in my mind as to whether I had made the right decision. Should I have picked some other area of medical practice to use my talents?

The phone rang about 2:30 AM early one morning and the emergency room supervisor at St. Francis Hospital alerted me to the admission of an elderly male patient with a severe nose bleed. The interne had tried packing the nose but the flow of blood continued. There was no question posterior packing was needed.

I could hear the wind howling as I left the house. The chill factor must have been about 20 degrees below zero. The weather was typical of a February night in New England. This kind of atmospheric condition seemed to precipitate nosebleeds in the elderly for some reason. Just as I was about to enter the garage I heard the phone ring again. This time it was the City Hospital which later became known as McCook. This was a hospital established primarily for the care of the indigent. I had been accepted as a member of the staff during my first years in private practice.

After I answered the phone I realized I had a real dilemma. The patient at the City Hospital was a two-year-old child choking from smoke inhalation. I immediately sensed the child's problem was much more urgent.

I called the ER at the St. Francis Hospital and told the supervising nurse to have the nosebleed patient cross-matched and transfused. I also suggested she should have the ER interne reinforce the nasal packing. I knew that patient would survive the loss of some blood especially with a transfusion running, but a blocked airway in an infant requires immediate surgery if the baby is to survive.

As I pulled out of the driveway and turned on the heater, I couldn't help noticing the darkened houses of my neighbors. These were the homes of contractors, insurance executives, bankers, and other business people whose day began at 9 AM and ended at 5 PM. For a fleeting moment I was just a bit envious of them with their short work day and their uninterrupted nights.

I rounded the corner of my street and quickly entered the main road. There wasn't a flicker of headlights in any direction. At this hour who would be out traveling unless they were also on an errand of mercy or involved in some nefarious activity. Just as I reached the nearby intersection the traffic light turned red. I paused for a moment and saw no other vehicles in sight. I jammed my foot on the accelerator and jumped ahead through the beaming red light.

The City Hospital was about four miles away. I could easily reach it within five minutes. That would probably give me enough time to perform the tracheotomy and establish an airway before complete obstruction of the breathing occurred. Suddenly as I sped down the highway I became aware of a flashing light far behind me. Despite continuing my same speed the headlights of the pursuing car came closer.

Then, as I expected, the sound of a siren pierced the cold night air. I continued on without slowing down but the cop in the cruiser wasn't giving up. In a few moments the car with the town police emblem on the door pulled up beside me as I came to a stop.

With the physician's cross on my car I was annoyed by the delay on what was an emergency call and an errand of mercy. I resented the officer's questioning even more as he stood by my car door and appeared to be in no great hurry.

"Where do you think you're going?" he asked gruffly.

"I'm on my way to the hospital," I replied, trying to keep a civil tongue in my head.

"And what hospital are you going to?" he continued. It was getting to be like a third degree.

"The City Hospital," I yelled back at him, raising the decibel considerably. I was really starting to boil as he went on with his interrogation, apparently by the book. At no time did he say, "Follow me," as I half-expected him to say in his best policeman's manner.

"And why are you going there, may I ask?"

He slowed down his speech to arouse my temper and it worked exceptionally well.

"I have an emergency," I blasted back at him.

He was sounding more and more like an abrasive attorney in a movie court trial and I was becoming more and more irritated.

"What kind of emergency?" he said without batting an eyelash.

That was enough for me. I turned on him with both barrels.

"I'll be damned if I'm going to sit here answering your stupid questions while a child is struggling for her life at the hospital."

With that last statement I released the brake and zoomed ahead, leaving him standing there with his mouth still open. The hospital was still a few miles away and the officer followed me all the way despite my speed.

I had lost valuable time. I pulled up in front of the hospital, jumped out of the car and dashed through the emergency room door. Without stopping for a second I ran to the elevator, closed the metal gate, and left the policeman pounding on the outside.

Within a few moments I was in the operating room and checked the patient. There was no question about it, immediate surgery was necessary.

Without losing a second I changed into a scrub suit and did the indicated tracheotomy on the little two-year-old black girl. What a beautiful thing it was to see her breathing return to normal. She no longer gasped for air and her pale blue lips quickly regained a normal pink color. She was out of danger. I knew she would recover.

I applied a dressing to the wound. The OR supervisor came into the room and waited until I was done. She tapped me on the shoulder and I turned to her.

"I just wanted to let you know," she said smiling, "that a police officer came by and asked if you were really here for an emergency. I told him what you were doing and he left."

This incident occurred early in my practice and I never encountered any difficulties with the town police in the years following. Perhaps I was more careful or maybe there was instant recognition as there seems to be with obstetricians that the speeding doctor at 3 AM is usually performing his duties just like the police officers are.

I left the City Hospital and drove at a reasonable speed to the St. Francis Hospital located about a mile away. The bleeding patient was still oozing a small amount of blood from his nose but his condition was stable. I put in a posterior pack which stopped the bleeding immediately and then admitted him for further observation.

I returned home feeling great. I didn't even notice the darkened houses all around me. I had a glow that couldn't be extinguished. I took a short nap before starting another day. A good hot shower and a quick breakfast and I was fully refreshed. It had been a busy night. In the final analysis two patients recovered from their problems and that is the real reward in evaluating success or failure.

KIDS

Kids are Funny — Sometimes

"Anybody who hates kids and dogs can't be all that bad."

This aphorism attributed to W. C. Fields wouldn't meet with the approval of pediatricians and most physicians.

The quotation has been repeated so often that it has been accepted at times as gospel truth. It is acknowledged that the comedian made the statement, but primarily to get a laugh which it did. Those of us who have brought up children and included youngsters in our medical practice will sometimes agree with W. C. Fields. The little folk can be both exasperating and nerve-wracking, yet they bring a joy and a spark to our lives that nobody in his right mind would want to extinguish.

Each generation sprouts a new breed that often amazes those who precede them. As civilization goes on we do find that those who succeed us are making life more comfortable and lasting than those who lived before us.

In the practice of medicine we can recall fleetingly some of the anxious and distressing moments that were experienced when a youngster got out of hand and on a few occasions the frustrations brought on by the uncooperative parent.

Over the years it has been recognized and accepted that pediatricians have always been at the lowest end of the medical ladder economically. I cannot recall meeting or knowing of any child doctor who switched to another specialty. There is a certain love and affection for these little patients that makes financial return of strictly minor importance.

Unhappy Michael

He was a fair-haired five-year-old with a round, freckled face, but in obvious pain. His mother practically dragged him into the treatment room at the Brooklyn Eye and Ear Hospital.

"Michael has been crying with an earache since early this morning," his mother explained as she sat him down on the treatment chair.

"Did he have a sore throat or a cold before this happened," I asked.

"He had a runny nose for a few days, but he never gets sick. We came from Ireland three months ago and he misses his cousins and friends. I gave him an aspirin but he's been screeching with the pain for the past hour."

Michael's sobbing increased as I sat on the stool facing him. He eyed me with distrust as I prepared to examine him.

"Let me see how your throat is first, Michael, and then we'll look at your ear."

The throat showed normal-appearing tonsils but the left ear drum was reddened and swollen.

"Michael does have a bad infection of his ear, but we can give him some medicine to take care of it. He will have some pain for a few days."

"Thank you, Doctor. My husband is training to become a policeman like his uncle and he is away all day. It is difficult for us with few friends in Brooklyn where we live."

After examining my little patient I made an attempt to divert his attention from the discomfort in his ear.

"Do you go to school, Michael?" I asked gently.

There was no response except an increase in sobbing.

"What's your teacher's name, Michael?"

This too brought a blank response.

"Do you like living in America, Michael?"

This was certainly not the right question. Michael grabbed his mother's hand tightly and his screams of pain became louder.

After writing out the prescriptions for the infection and pain, I decided to make one final overture to win his friendship and perhaps lessen his discomfort. It was December 22nd and I was sure that this last attempt would win him over.

"Michael, soon it will be Christmas. Santa Claus will be coming to see you and you'll be getting lots of presents. Won't that make you happy?"

His response was immediate and somewhat unexpected. He rose from the chair, stopped sobbing, and stood before me almost defiantly and cried out, "Shit Christmas, shit Santa Claus, and shit you, Doctor."

With that he dashed out of the room toward the clinic exit followed by his apologizing and embarrassed mother.

So much for a child's view of the adult world.

"I Wanna Go Home"

Little Maria was no different from most of the children admitted for tonsil surgery. She was frightened as she came off the elevator screaming, "I wanna go home."

As a first-year resident on the ENT service of the Brooklyn Eye and Ear, one of my responsibilities was putting the patient to sleep in preparation for tonsil surgery. The anesthesia of choice was ether, which was a harsh induction agent, but one of the safest anesthetics available at that time.

Children responded somewhat violently to this procedure and that was understandable. In those days the youngster was brought from the safety of his bed and carried on a stretcher to the strange environment of the induction room which was reeking with the unpleasant smelling fumes of ether. My last patient of the morning could be heard crying and screaming as soon as she entered the area.

"I wanna go home," she kept repeating as I approached her with the can of ether and mask in my hands. It took several nurses to hold the patient down, but despite the security straps she continued to struggle. When she stopped her anguished screams for a moment, I started a conversation with her.

"What is your name?" I asked.

"Maria," she replied. "I wanna go home."

"How old are you, Maria?"

"Eight years old. I wanna go home."

"Do you go to school?"

"Yes. I wanna go home."

"What grade are you in, Maria?"

"Thoid grade. I wanna go home."

"Can you say third grade?"

"Yes, thoid grade. I wanna go home."

"Where do you live, Maria?"

"Greenpernt. I wanna go home."

"Can you say Greenpoint ?"

"Yes. Greenpernt. I wanna go home."

As I placed the mask over her face and started to pour the ether, she grabbed the mask and pushed it aside.

"If you don't let me go, I'll piss my pants," she threatened.

She did just that just as I replaced the mask and restarted the anesthetic.

Preparations for surgery, as well as the anesthetic used, have undergone great changes since those days. Although the anesthetic that was administered did prevent the patient from suffering pain, there had to be a huge psychological trauma. It was due to our failure to recognize the need for proper preparation prior to surgery that is so important for children.

"Hey Mom, This Doctor's Been Drinking"

My first patient was seven-year-old Eric. As I proceeded to examine him, he pulled back and yelled to his mother sitting close by.

"Hey mom, this doctor's been drinking. I can smell whiskey."

I had just spent a good part of the morning in the operating room with a heavy schedule of tonsil operations. Immediately after surgery I hurried off to the office where Eric was my first patient.

I must admit that in those first years of practice many tonsillectomies were performed by the members of the ENT department. There was no such thing as an antibiotic to cut down recurrent throat infections. The only effective deterrent to days in bed and loss of school attendance was a T & A (tonsillectomy and adenoidectomy). The alternative, recommended by a few physicians, was simply bed rest and aspirin. This regimen could result in cardiac and kidney complications and therefore was not always a suitable choice.

While sitting behind the patient during tonsil surgery, the fumes from the ether anesthetic were gradually absorbed by the operator into his breathing passages, his skin and the clothes under his operating suit. Occasionally I would be aware of sniffing or comments from individuals with whom I might be in close contact. This might occur in a small retail store where customers are clustered together around the counter. The same thing would happen in a crowded elevator where there were always quizzical looks and a little sniffing. Some people would even comment, "This place smells like a hospital."

After hearing Eric's impression of the smell and finishing my examination, I took the mother aside and described the condition of his throat and ears and recommended the proper treatment.

"I am concerned by Eric's saying he thought he smelled whiskey. The odor, which you probably have also noted, comes from the ether anesthesia to which I am exposed during my tonsil surgeries each morning. I can't understand why this ether smell makes Eric think I've been drinking."

"Doctor," Eric's mother replied. "My husband is an alcoholic. When he drinks to excess he becomes abusive. Eric has become aware of his father's drinking on those occasions. I guess he can smell the strong odor of whiskey. Apparently the ether smell makes him think of his father, who often strikes him and me too, when he's drunk. I'll explain to him that you haven't been drinking and the source of that odor."

Eric was seen on several more occasions after his first visit, but these examinations weren't after a morning of tonsillectomies. He said nothing further about smelling whiskey and he showed no reluctance in being examined.

Despite a shower after finishing my operative schedule, apparently this didn't completely remove the ether scent, although it appeared to minimize it to some degree. I was happy, however, when the new anesthetics eliminated the need for ether and allowed me to face the public without any questioning looks as I stood next to them.

Stripping the Christmas Tree

"Don't take those ornaments off the tree."

My secretary, Anne Murray, had spent many hours decorating the Christmas tree with tinsel and dozens of the delicate bulbs. She took justifiable pride in her work of art, but the two youngsters, age four and six, saw the colorful pieces of hanging art in a different light.

When the two young boys first entered the waiting room, their hyperactivity was restricted to somersaults. This caused some annoyance to the other patients, but not to their father who said nothing. Then the brilliance of the Christmas tree caught their attention.

They proceeded to remove a few of the bulbs and began tossing them back and forth.

"Here, Jimmy, catch mine."

"No, Bobby, you catch mine."

After a few missed catches, Anne came out of her office and told them not to touch the ornaments which she replaced on the tree. Their father continued to sit unperturbed reading a magazine.

They remained quiet for several minutes and then renewed the ball game. Anne said nothing until she heard the crash of the ornaments. She retrieved the pieces and at the same time admonished the children.

"Now look what you've done after I told you not to play with those pretty ornaments."

As she returned to her office cubicle, the father rose from his chair and walked to the office window. He was over six-feet tall and had a booming voice. Back at his workshop, he told my secretary, people called him Tex because he moved from Texas three years ago. He now addressed Anne in a voice loud enough so all the others in the waiting room could hear him clearly.

"You don't like kids, do you?"

With that statement he turned and walked back to his chair to renew his reading. At the same time the two children decided to renew their ball game.

It was too much for Anne who came into the treatment room with tears in her eyes.

"I tried to tell them in a nice way," she said, "that they should sit down and read the comic books, but they just won't behave no matter what I say."

"Anne, we have one room unoccupied back here. Bring them in and I will take care of them right away."

Their examination was completed without incident and a follow-up visit was not needed until after the Christmas season. I found that it was better to see some children as soon as they entered the office. It saved a lot of wear-and-tear on me, the office staff, and especially the office furnishings.

7

THE MEDIA

Fatal Advice from a Medical Columnist

"If your youngster has croup, don't rush him off to the emergency room and have a quack specialist give him a shot of adrenalin. Just hang him over an open window sill and allow the cool refreshing breeze to open up his breathing passages."

Dr. Brady, a medical columnist whose advice appeared in a Hartford newspaper, made this recommendation to his readers one week before I was called to see a patient with severe difficulty in breathing. The call from the emergency room was most urgent and occurred on a cold wintry night in December.

"Please come quickly, Doctor. We have just admitted a three-year-old child who has had croup all day and is barely breathing. Please hurry."

Although I dressed quickly and arrived at the hospital within minutes, the child was already lifeless and resuscitation efforts were unsuccessful. The patient's history indicated he had croup and the autopsy findings confirmed this diagnosis.

One week later I received another call to see a second youngster who was severely cyanotic by the time the parents brought him to the hospital. I immediately performed a tracheotomy in the emergency room which restored his breathing and in spite of the child's condition when he was first seen, he survived.

After learning that the parents of both youngsters had followed Dr. Brady's advice in the newspaper I wrote to the editor of the paper.

"In the past week I have seen two children in the emergency room of the St. Francis Hospital. Each youngster had the croup which should have indicated a call to the family doctor. The parents admitted they had delayed contacting their physicians because they had tried Dr. Brady's suggested treatment for croup they had read in your paper. The first child died shortly after his arrival at the hospital. The second child was more fortunate. An emergency tracheotomy that saved his life was performed in the emergency room as soon as he was seen.

"In his column Dr. Brady wrote that the quack specialist in the emergency room would only give the youngster a shot of adrenalin. I am not a quack specialist and I don't use adrenalin to treat croup. Furthermore, I don't agree with his statement that advises the parent to open the window and hang the child's head over the sill to breathe in the fresh air. A child's life is very precious to the parents and the physician who becomes responsible for his care. It is absolutely ludicrous for a medical columnist to recommend advice that can be fatal as happened in this case. At no point did Dr Brady advise that the patient's physician be contacted in this life-threatening disease."

My letter wasn't published, but in reply the editor attempted to defend Brady's column by stating that all of Brady's articles are reviewed by an editorial board before publication.

Being of a cantankerous nature, I replied to the editor: "Please list the names of the doctors who make up the editorial board."

Further correspondence revealed there was absolutely no medical supervision of Dr. Brady's columns.

Not being content to let sleeping dogs lie, I contacted a fellow otolaryngologist, Dr. Lester Coleman, an active practitioner in New York City. Dr. Coleman also wrote a medical column published in many newspapers throughout the country. I had made his acquaintance at a national ENT meeting a year earlier.

A detailed description of my correspondence and Dr. Brady's column were sent to Dr. Coleman. He immediately dispatched a letter to the editor of the paper protesting its failure to publish my correspondence. It all ended up in a complete stalemate. Dr. Coleman was told he wasn't aware of the facts in the case and therefore was not in a position to make any judgements.

During this written confrontation through the mail, I contacted the Director of the Hartford County Medical Association. Joe Gordon informed me that the medical association had been trying to curtail Dr. Brady's column for years. Their suggestion for a bona fide medical evaluation of his articles was completely ignored.

Apparently Dr. Brady was untouchable because of his popularity. His recommendations were followed religiously by readers throughout the country. He had a folksy type of presentation that appealed to the general reading public. It was the same approach he used for his patients when he practiced in a tiny Pennsylvania hamlet. His written medical advice had spread from a small weekly news periodical to a national syndicated column in a brief period of time. A good number of his writings included common-sense suggestions for the treatment of the common cold, which he referred to as "CRI" (common respiratory inflammation), and the relief of painful joints due to arthritis with aspirin and calcium.

He often included some of the correspondence from his devoted readers. One faithful disciple wrote: " My son swallowed a whistle and I haven't heard nothing from it. What shall I do?" Dr. Brady had these comforting words: "This too will pass."

Sometimes his recommendations were laughable and ridiculous. "If you swallow a denture use the suggestion of a dentist from Worcester, Massachusetts. Take two inches of unraveled threads and swallow them with teaspoonfuls of applesauce. This will form a cocoon around the denture allowing the dental piece to pass through the intestine without difficulty."

It was a short time after this column appeared that a prominent Hartford citizen was admitted to the hospital after swallowing his partial denture. He was observed for several days with x-rays taken regularly as the denture delayed its descent from the stomach into the duodenum and then into the colon. Three days later the patient developed some abdominal pain and x-rays showed the denture caught in the lower intestinal tract. The surgeons were now forced to remove the dental piece through an extensive abdominal incision.

There wasn't any report as to whether the applesauce-and-thread treatment was tried or suggested. The major operation and prolonged hospitalization could probably have been avoided simply by having the patient undergo endoscopy. Such a procedure could have removed the denture with the esophagoscope on the day of admission.

The medical columns now written in most major newspapers are composed by very knowledgeable physicians. The Hartford Courant and other leading newspapers use their pages to bring their readers up to date with well-documented medical information. Not only the reading public, but even the practicing physician may gain some valuable insight when he reviews some of these published presentations. Television gives constant update on the latest treatments in various diseases and usually these commentaries are supported by experts in the involved field. The access to medical knowledge has now been expanded to the Internet. But be careful, the modern version of the snake-oil medicine man may have given up his horse and buggy, but you still might find him lurking behind that screen.

"Caveat emptor: Let the buyer beware."

A Call from Mike Wallace of "60 Minutes"

"Hello, this is Mike Wallace speaking. I understand you charge a fee for admitting a patient to the hospital."

When my young associate received this call he was naturally mystified by the statement. He asked Wallace to get in touch with him the next day so that the specific patient's records could be reviewed. Prior to the follow-up call, my associate and I went over the chart of the individual named by Wallace. The patient had been seen several months earlier because of a chronic ear condition. Office treatment by my associate failed to control the drainage and surgery was advised.

Following admission to the hospital, routine blood and urine tests as well as chest x-rays were ordered as part of the preoperative studies. The chest films revealed the presence of active tuberculosis and the scheduled mastoidectomy was canceled. Consultation with a chest specialist was obtained followed by arranging the patient's transfer to a TB sanitarium. All of this was done by my associate who did the additional paper work since he had arranged for the patient's admission. Because all of this required considerable time and effort, a charge of $25 was placed on his bill for the workup involved. There wasn't any indication this reasonable billing wouldn't be accepted. For some unknown reason the patient decided to bring this to the attention of Mike Wallace. In those early days of the "60 Minutes" program, Wallace was apparently doing a lot of legwork while gathering information for the show.

When we reviewed the billing charges we noted that the secretary, as in all hospitalizations, had also recorded the hospital admission date. This date was followed by the notation "admission for surgery." No surgery was performed, but on the date of discharge three days later the charge of $25 was posted.

When Mike Wallace called the next day, I identified myself as an associate of our group and explained the reason for the charge. The conversation ended immediately and we heard no more from "60 Minutes" or Mike Wallace.

On occasion when watching "60 Minutes" I often listen with a sense of doubt and refuse to accept the information that is presented as gospel truth. From my brief experience it seemed that Mike Wallace was willing to sacrifice the professional reputation of innocent physicians.

However he didn't hesitate to pander to a patient who should have been grateful for a doctor who made a critical diagnosis and arranged proper treatment that probably saved his life and the lives of people with whom he associated.

During my years of practice I tried to avoid confrontation whenever possible. At times conflicting opinions occurred and it was often sensible to say nothing and just back away. On occasion, however, it was necessary to take a stand whenever an important principle was involved.

John Stuart Mill, the English philosopher, stated "Actions are right in proportion as they tend to promote happiness, wrong as they tend to promote the reverse of happiness."

Many very fine physicians with whom I was acquainted were well-respected for their ability and their honesty. It was disturbing at times when a controversial issue developed and they refused to be vocal on one side or the other. Looking back I realize that their silence enhanced their reputation as peacemakers. However, it was upsetting to me that a firmer resistance was not taken when these doctors were aware of what was detrimental to the care of patients and even turned away from an attack on their own personal philosophy.

It's always easier to say nothing and it certainly makes life more comfortable if you don't interfere and become involved in the fray. Having fought my way through my early years in order to survive, it had become a natural instinct to take up the sword in defense of principles. Sometimes the odds were overwhelmingly against me and I should have pulled back, but that little thing called conscience forced me into action no matter what the cost.

Opposing certain actions of the media sometimes resulted in lengthy and frustrating confrontations. Not everyone agreed that I was acting properly in taking stands against the behemoths of the industry with overwhelming odds against success.

8
PERSONAL ILLNESSES

Dizziness

"Do you feel alright, Doctor?"

The operating room nurse came over to my side as I started to rise from the stool and then quickly sat down. My last surgical case, a four-hour mastoid operation, had just been finished. Suddenly I noted a severe ringing in my ears with a marked unsteadiness I had never experienced before. I grabbed onto the side of the operating table to keep from falling as a cold clammy sweat and a feeling of nausea overwhelmed me.

The nurses who had scrubbed on the mastoid case quickly recognized my distress and came around to assist me. Nora Walsh, the head supervisor, was called and came on the run. She insisted on guiding me down to the doctors' lounge.

"You'd better lie down before you fall down," Nora said.

This was a command from the supervisor and I did what I was told. Once I lay back on the couch the nausea disappeared, but the room was still spinning around.

After a few minutes I was able to assure Miss Walsh that the crisis was over.

"Don't worry," I said. "The worst has passed, but I think I'll stay here for a few minutes before getting dressed."

Lying back on the couch allowed me to do a self-assessment of my problem. With the ringing in my ears and a definite loss of hearing which I now noticed, there was no doubt in my mind that my symptoms of vertigo were typical of Meniere's disease.

Other possibilities would have to be considered, including tumors of the eight cranial nerve which controls hearing and equilibrium. Recently some published articles had indicated that very often the likelihood of tumor hadn't been considered seriously when dizziness occurred. The development of newer X-ray techniques in recent years has helped to diagnose these growths much earlier.

Dizziness is one of the more common symptoms encountered in

any ENT practice. The unsteadiness is frequently accompanied by ringing in the ears, which is called tinnitus. The attack often comes on without warning while driving the car, walking down stairs, or enjoying the company of friends.

A diagnosis of Meniere's is usually made by the physician when a patient is first seen with the triad of symptoms as described. However, a little knowledge is a bad thing and I must confess that the possibility of an eight-nerve tumor was one of the diagnostic possibilities that lurked in the back of my mind.

When I began to feel better, I called my office and canceled all my appointments for the day. I then put in a call to an internist friend, Dr. Franco. I explained my problem and asked him to check me out.

He told me to come in immediately. He skipped his lunch and gave me a complete physical examination. This was essentially negative except for a slight unsteadiness which I noted when I stood with my eyes closed. This usually is present when there is a disturbance of the labyrinth and is typical of Meniere's disease.

A skull x-ray was negative. Actually such x-rays in those years were usually of little value unless the tumor was far advanced. Nowadays, with C.A.T. scans and other specialized techniques, even the smallest growths can be detected in the early stages.

I then checked with Dr. O'Hurley, an otologist in my department. He also arranged to see me immediately. His examination, including a complete hearing evaluation, was also essentially negative except for the slight bilateral hearing loss I had for several years. This was now accentuated in the left ear where most of the tinnitus was located.

Because of our concern about a possible eight-nerve tumor, we both agreed that a consultation with Dr. Schucknecht was advisable. This internationally-known and respected otologist was the head of the ear department at the Massachusetts Eye and Ear Infirmary. I had become acquainted with him early in my practice. Within two days of my call he graciously received me in his office.

Before his examination he reviewed my history.

"Have you had any similar episodes of dizziness?" he asked.

"Not since I went overseas on an L.S.T., a flat-bottomed ship that rolled with every wave," I said.

"Have you been feeling unusually fatigued lately?" he continued.

"Not that morning, but I had been more tired at the end of the day for several weeks."

"How do you account for that?" he said.

"Probably because I'd been taking an advanced course in nasal plastic surgery."

I explained to Dr. Schucknecht that these were surgical anatomy sessions given in New York primarily for nose and throat specialists.

"The course was held on Tuesday and Thursday evenings from 7 PM to 10 PM. I closed my office at 2:30 in the afternoon and drove to New Haven. There I took the 4:00 PM train to New York arriving just when the teaching started. The return trip by the 11 PM train brought me to New Haven usually by 1:30 AM. The drive back home got me to bed by 2:30 in the morning."

Dr. Schucknecht and I agreed that this could be a very tiring routine, especially when I had an operating schedule starting at 8 AM and lasting till noon. By the time I finished rounds it was time for a quick lunch and hectic office appointments in the afternoon. There was no question that I was stretching my youthful enthusiasm to the breaking point.

The otological examination by Dr. Schucknecht included a caloric test which involves injecting cold water into each ear and watching the eye movements for any abnormal reaction. Further testing of my hearing was done, as well as a more detailed evaluation of the ear by x-ray. This radiological exam gave a much better identification of the inner ear because of the advanced equipment at the Eye and Ear Infirmary. This study showed no evidence of a tumor.

After completion of all the tests, Dr. Schucknecht was most reassuring as he explained that the tests confirmed that this was a true Meniere's attack. Except for the use of nicotinic acid, which does seem to help in some cases, no other medication was advised. The restriction of fluids and salt was also suggested and this again has been universally recommended but not guaranteed to help all patients.

When a doctor is a patient, it is important to be completely objective and in most cases have your attending physician make the decisions for you. I had complete faith in Dr. Schucknecht and such confidence helped to effect an improvement. His experience in dealing with such symptoms gave me the reassuring comfort I needed.

After the evaluation of my condition, I resumed my operative schedule as well as my office appointments. The mild unsteadiness which had persisted for some time gradually disappeared completely.

A physician doesn't need to have all the diseases experienced by patients to be able to treat them adequately and successfully. However, after developing and being evaluated for my own symptoms, I felt I had a better approach to such problems. I found that I could empathize much more completely with those who presented themselves with a complaint of dizziness.

During my years of practice I was fortunate in escaping any serious illnesses, although there were a few scares. Except for the usual minor colds and aches and pains, I turned to physicians whose expertise I trusted whenever a distressing symptom affected me. There is one dictum that has been passed down from one generation of physicians to the next: "The doctor who treats himself has a fool for a patient."

I have tried to follow that advice.

Diagnosis: Metastatic Carcinoma

"It doesn't look good."

The words of the radiologist were ominous, to say the least, as he pointed to a suspicious shadow on my chest film that had just been developed. At first I couldn't believe the spot, clearly seen on my left lung, represented anything that might be life-threatening.

"Do you think it might be a defect on the film?" I suggested to Dr. Cobb as he examined the x-ray with me. Such markings are called artifacts which are changes caused by processing and subsequent films will show a normal-appearing lung.

"Dick," I said, "I'm not a smoker and we all know shadows like this mean cancer and are found in patients who are heavy smokers."

When I was ten my mother saw me puffing away in front of the mirror. She strongly advised me not to do it again, reinforcing her admonition with a strong tap on the backside.

Dr. Cobb now had another suggestion.

"Let's take a look at your lungs with the fluoroscope," he said.

He saw the same lesion and it was definitely not a shadow caused by a blood vessel or old scarring from some previous unknown inflammation.

"I'm going to take another set of films," he said, "just to be doubly sure that these findings are correct."

He was looking for any possible technical error that could change the diagnosis, but the results were the same.

One advantage in being a physician patient is that there is no communication gap. You call upon a consultant whom you know is qualified, but also a good friend. It tends to make the presentation of a serious diagnosis easier to accept. The difficulty in being a doctor and a patient is that a little knowledge can be a dangerous thing. You have a wider appreciation of what the diagnosis and the prognosis might mean. The whole future of your life, your family, and your medical career become more immediately apparent.

Sometimes the spots found on a chest film are readily identified as inflammatory and therefore not malignant. This coin-sized lesion didn't have the same outline as that found in an infection. It was very possible that I was harboring a tumor that could be life-threatening. Dr. Cobb and I agreed that it would be wise to have further medical consultation and advice as to how to proceed.

The chest x-ray was part of the annual physical examination I decided upon several years earlier, when I encountered the distressing dizzy spell that sent me hurrying off for a medical evaluation and ear consultation. The most recent physical exam by my internist was completely normal and had been done just the day before the x-ray. That was the reason the x-ray findings were such a shocker.

After calling Dr. Franco, my internist, we decided on a consultation with the chest specialists the next day. I hoped their interpretation of the film along with my internist's recommendations would result in a mind-easing that could remove the psychic trauma that had developed.

My first thought was to postpone telling my wife about the x-rays until after I had seen the chest physicians. However, the 24 hours of concealing my own problems and destiny proved to be an uncomfortable strain. After dinner that night I confided to her exactly what I knew, that the x-rays showed a spot in the left lung and that my future, although not grim, was somewhat cloudy at best.

To compound the problem, I had received a letter three days earlier from a young doctor on the west coast. He had decided to accept the offer of association with me. He had already sold his house and was planning on joining my practice in ten more weeks. At this point in time I wasn't too sure I'd still be alive.

A surgeon friend, Dr. Morris, had visited my office shortly before my chest x-ray. A recurrent wax problem was causing some annoying blockage of his hearing. He had been diagnosed with cancer of the lung two months earlier. During that time he had lost such a tremendous amount of weight that I barely recognized him as he sat in the treatment chair. It's not uncommon for a physician to encounter patients with a progressive disease that ends fatally. Suddenly it seemed that I was facing the same reality.

After the combined consultation with the chest specialists and my internist, I was no nearer a resolution of my difficulties than I had been before.

Dr. Lahiri and Dr. Godar, both excellent pulmonary specialists, reviewed the films while I sat beside them.

They began to ask questions.

"Where have you visited in the past year? There are several common inflammations that could show up on chest films as shadows on the lungs. These include fungus infections that can be acquired during travel."

"I was in Mexico for a medical meeting one year ago," I said, "but I wasn't sick while there or since that time."

Several tests for fungi were ordered and these were all negative. In addition a tuberculin test was done and this was positive. Having grown up in Boston, this test had been done several times before and it was always positive, which is not uncommon in those residing in large metropolitan cities.

One recommendation suggested by my consultants was an examination of the lungs by bronchoscopy. This procedure could obtain tissue leading to a positive diagnosis as to the cause of the x-ray shadow. Some years of personal experience in performing bronchoscopies prompted me to turn down that suggested procedure. The density on the chest film was on the periphery of the lung and there was no way that a bronchoscope could reach that area.

Dr. Franco now made another suggestion.

"The only way we can determine the cause is by an exploration of the chest and if necessary take a biopsy."

I made a quick response to that.

"Such a procedure," I said, "would end up with the removal of part of the lung for examination. That is a major operation for a possible inflammatory lesion."

Nothing more was said about doing chest surgery.

The pulmonary physicians then suggested a waiting period of one week and then a series of chest films called laminograms. These pictures would give an in-depth outline of the shadow and possibly help in identifying the mass in case it was malignant.

Before this second set of x-rays was done, I learned about a biopsy procedure being done at the Johns Hopkins Medical Center in Baltimore. With special fluoroscopic equipment guiding them the surgeons at that hospital could perform a biopsy of the lung under local anesthesia. In essence, this was a needle biopsy. This appealed to me since it wouldn't require the chest to be opened up. If the tissue report from that type of biopsy was negative, I could be back to work the next day. I decided to wait on the results of the laminograms before considering any further procedures.

The chest physicians were most supportive and agreed with my decision to forego any operation. They were as puzzled as my internist in trying to determine the cause of the lung shadow, but they were also anxious to establish a definite diagnosis.

Part of the decision-making had to rest with me. This is true whether the patient is a physician or a lay person with no medical knowledge. When the diagnosis is definite and life-threatening then the patient should always abide by his doctor's recommendations. Since there was uncertainty about the cause in my case, it was up to me to make the final decision.

In the second week of my evaluations, I again visited Dr. Cobb's office. In addition to being an excellent radiologist, he had a good sense of humor and a very supportive manner. He and his office staff were also most cooperative in fitting me into their busy schedule so that it wouldn't interfere with my own office appointments. I had definitely decided that as long as I was asymptomatic, without either fever or fatigue, that there wouldn't be any change in my practice routine.

For years a vegetable garden in the rear of my home had been my pride and joy. When I was hit with the diagnosis of a possible lung cancer, I decided to spend more free time working the soil. The garden area was purposely enlarged from 20 by 30 feet to a space measuring about 40 by 50. The harvest was much more than my family could handle, but I made a lot of friends happy by sharing the crop.

Completion of the laminograms in the second week was a crushing blow and added to the mental stress which I found difficult to control. The original films showed a shadow in the upper part of my left lung, but now there was a density in the middle of my right lung. My disease, whatever it was, had spread to the opposite side. This made the future look more ominous than ever, since the tumor, if cancerous, had probably come from some other organ in my body and was now metastasizing.

My internist now advised hospitalization since multiple tests, including more x-rays, were indicated to determine where the possible primary cancer was located.

Hospitalization was one suggestion that I strongly vetoed. Being cooped up in the hospital and having different tests performed each day for a week or more would only increase my anxiety. I felt that all examinations could be done on an outpatient basis without disrupting my practice. I was anxious to avoid any brooding which I was sure to experience while lying around in a four-walled hospital room.

A few days after the laminograms were done, Dr. Cobb took all the films to a seminar of some fifty radiologists who were meeting in New Haven. The opinions were just about evenly divided between those who thought it was cancer and those who voted for a diagnosis of a nonmalignant inflammation.

One morning while making rounds at the hospital, I stopped Dr. Fox, a urologist and a good friend.

"Brendan," I said, I have a problem that requires consultation."

After I explained the results of the x-rays, Dr. Fox agreed that a simple urological examination could be done with further cystoscopic evaluation if indicated.

"Your only concern would probably be the prostate and the testes," he said.

After he checked them he said, "Both your prostate and testes are perfectly normal and not a likely cause of the x-ray shadows."

This response by Dr. Fox was reassuring and I continued on my rounds.

A few days later I met Dr. Burns while he was checking his patients on the surgical ward.

"John," I said, "I have a small mole on my right thigh. Would you check it with a biopsy to make sure it's not a melanoma."

I explained to Dr. Burns the reason for my inquiry. He immediately had a small surgical set made up and under local anesthesia excised the mole. It was benign.

Many years earlier my mother had developed a melanoma on her leg that metastasized to the groin. However, she succumbed to a brain hemorrhage unrelated to the melanoma.

About the fourth week I noted a discoloration under the nail of my left big toe. This had been present for several weeks and I knew that malignant melanomas had been reported as sometimes occurring under the nails of the toes and fingers. I decided my fears were unfounded and that the discoloration probably developed from stubbing my toe. It disappeared within a few weeks.

Wednesday morning was my regular day at the x-ray office for additional chest films. X-rays of other organs were also taken in an effort to determine where the lesions in my lungs might have had their origin. On the third week Dr. Cobb noticed additional densities on both lungs, which of course caused me a great deal of worry.

Along with the chest films Dr. Franco ordered x-rays of my long bones which frequently will show evidence of metastases if cancer is present. All of these were normal.

The fourth week included a number of x-rays which proved to be somewhat uncomfortable but we all agreed were necessary. Gastrointestinal and gallbladder series were also negative. After the gallbladder series Dr. Cobb had a word of warning for me.

"The dye we use has a strong cathartic effect," he said, "usually within a few hours."

Late that morning while on my way to the golf course for a tournament, the dye caught up with me. I returned home for a quick change of trousers. The episode proved to be a real stimulus to my golf game since I was rewarded with the best score I ever had. However, I don't recommend that as a method to improve your game.

At one time during the course of all these examinations, the suggestion was made that a course of antibiotics should be given for a possible infectious disease. Since there weren't any symptoms of malaise or fever and the blood and urine examinations were normal, we finally agreed that no medication was needed.

During these weeks I didn't have any of the expected symptoms of cough or chest pain, although the x-rays continued to show an increase in the number of densities in my lungs. All of my consultants scratched their heads wondering what was going on in my chest. They had no idea as to what was happening and naturally I shared their quandary. Being a physician as well as a patient caused me to recall the sage reflection that a little knowledge can be a bad thing. I was in a constant state of mental turmoil.

The chest x-rays on the fifth week gave the first sign of hope that I was improving.

Several of the densities appeared to be smaller. However the view of the left lung showed another shadow not previously observed. Again Dr. Cobb brought the films from his office to the hospital so that all members of the x-ray staff could review them and offer an opinion. These specialists were encouraging in their agreement that the changes did show slight improvement.

We decided to omit any further x-rays until the seventh week. This would allow more time for improvement to take place. Up to this point all the other organs in my body had been tested for a possible source of a malignancy that could spread to the lungs. In each and every instance the results were completely negative.

The chest laminograms on the seventh week were a cause for cheering. The shadows in my left lung had completely disappeared and the densities on the right side were markedly diminished.

Dr. Cobb, always optimistic, was most reassuring as he exclaimed, "I think you are now out of the woods."

Several series of films were taken at two-week intervals and all showed improvement. On August 25th, thirteen weeks after my original x-rays, the final films were taken. There was no evidence of the lesions that had been scattered throughout my lungs in the series of films taken over the course of the previous three months.

I couldn't restrain my joy. All those who had been involved, including my personal physician, the consultants, and of course, my office staff, were just as thrilled as I was with the final report. The x-ray technicians had always been solicitous and supportive during my many weeks of examinations. I sent a case of champagne to their office and suggested they toast my victory.

In the practice of medicine some findings are unexpectedly discovered only because of the diversified technological procedures employed on routine evaluations or during the search for the cause of a mystifying disease.

Several years after my experience an article in one of the medical journals described the x-ray findings of multiple lung shadows in patients who were exposed to dogs with heartworm disease. The report stated that the chest x-rays had been ordered as part of yearly physical examinations and the unusual densities were noted in asymptomatic patients. This report had not been published at the time of my own problem.

I contacted a local veterinarian for his opinion. This very interested young man asked me a few pertinent questions.

"Before your x-ray findings," he asked, "did your dog become ill and require attention by a veterinarian."

"No," I answered, "but some months earlier he was coughing and gagging for several days. I made arrangements to take him to our hospital lab for a possible bronchoscopy and esophagoscopy, thinking that she might have a bone stuck in her throat. But her coughing cleared up on the second day so nothing was done."

The veterinarian laughed and said, "When did your dog die?"

"My dog is living and in good health," I replied.

"If your dog had heartworm disease she would have died within a few weeks after the onset of that canine illness. Therefore, the dog couldn't have been the source of your x-ray findings."

Undoubtedly, I had an asymptomatic viral infection that caused the chest x-ray changes without any other findings. If I hadn't decided on that annual physical examination, I might never have experienced those difficult weeks of worry which followed the x-ray report.

I wrote a brief description of my experience which was published in Medical Economics, a national magazine distributed to physicians.

My article, "Why I am against Annual Physical and X-ray Examinations," brought a number of comments, not all favorable. Some doctors pointed out the discovery of chest diseases that weren't suspected until a routine chest x-ray was done. I do agree with their arguments, but in my case it caused me several months of great concern.

Annual physicals can help bring out problems that haven't yet surfaced. But I remember the preface in Boyd's Pathology which was our bible in school:

"After performing many thousands of autopsies, I am astounded by the number of diseases in their organs about which patients had no complaint. The wonder is not that we die, but that we live as long as we do."

I agree with Boyd's observation.

The Power of Positive Thinking

A positive attitude is important in overcoming any problem. This is especially true when you are threatened with a serious or sometimes terminal illness. Norman Vincent Peale was one of the first to espouse the power of positive thinking.

Norman Cousins emphasized this in his "Anatomy of an Illness," written some years after I went through my traumatic episode. He had been given a very gloomy prognosis when he was attacked by a crippling illness. In spite of his doctor's predictions, he was able to overcome the disability and recovered completely. His story is not only fascinating, but should be required reading for anyone facing what appears to be a hopeless future.

Siegel in "Love, Medicine, and Miracles" repeats the same theme as Cousins. He includes the case histories of patients who were encouraged to believe they could live a long satisfying life despite the seriousness of their illness. Siegel stresses the use of support groups.

An endocrinologist, Dr. Deepak Chopra, writes in many of his books and teaches in his seminars that the mind is capable of controlling the body and even heal it of disease. The popularity of transcendental meditation is based on this same concept.

Dr. Steven Locke, a psychiatrist, believes that mental states do have an influence on the immune system. However, he has found no evidence that these changes in the immune system affect the disease process. Several years ago Dr. David Freeman wrote an interesting article, "Heal Thyself." He recounted the overpowering mental stress he endured during the months his wife was experiencing severe complications following major surgery. In the midst of these many many months of her near-death problems and her slow, agonizing recovery, he experienced a major depression. The emotional state that developed was compounded by various physical symptoms which he immediately self-diagnosed as heart attacks, malignancies, or brain tumors. With the help of his doctors, all of the symptoms disappeared except for the depression which persisted for many months and required psychiatric help.

Although I didn't experience the traumas to the psyche that struck Dr. Freeman, I can readily appreciate and understand all the sufferings that developed. One of the most important results of his illness was a greater empathy and sense of sharing with his patients' sicknesses and their tales of mental anguish.

I understand that fully and feel the same way.

Unfortunately, the new approach to treatment in medicine has brought on another breed of entrepreneurs who proclaim that they are the new messiahs. The danger is there may be a temptation by some to bypass the legitimate physician and his scientific approach by a vain attempt to encourage the patient to cure himself.

Holistic medicine has much to offer, but I'm totally opposed to any approach that doesn't include a proper evaluation by the patient's own personal physician. It's the doctor's responsibility to spend time with the patients and encourage them to engage themselves in a useful life in which they have many things to do. The time left, as with all of us, is known only to the Almighty.

Alternative treatments are now given widespread coverage in the press, radio, and television. Much of this has been fostered and heavily underwritten by groups or individuals who see the dollar sign waving before them. There is no question that much can be accomplished by seeking and using alternative approaches to treatment as I learned during my years of practice. Unfortunately, many of the entrepreneurs who are involved in so-called natural substances, herbal medicines, multivitamin therapies, mineral baths, and touch and aroma therapy are a modern copy of last century's traveling medicine man pitching his snake-oil preparations that will cure in one week every disease known to man.

FAITH AND HOPE

Following the death of my father there was never, to my recollection, any weeping or wailing in our household about the unkind fates that beset us. Often when we ran into any problems our mother reminded us that "the Lord fits the back to the burden."

The threat of any serious illness or catastrophe can be stressful and unsettling to the victim. A lot of support is needed from all sides and that includes family, friends, and clergy. In the case of a foreboding illness, the doctor should supply more than just the proper medical therapy.

In addition to the help and personal interest of concerned physicians, I was especially fortunate in having a very supportive office staff. Naturally they were aware of the undiagnosed lung densities which, week by week, not only failed to disappear, but in the first five or six weeks continued to pop up almost everywhere in my chest x-rays. The staff continued to work diligently while I carried out my duties in the office and the operating room.

Nowadays there is much discussion of endorphins, the group of proteins with potent opioid properties that occur naturally in the brain. These chemicals make you feel good and are said to increase one's ability to overcome severe stress. Perhaps I may have had a buildup of these endorphins, which along with my family and a deep religious faith, helped to carry me through a perilous journey.

There is much in the newspapers lately about the need for spiritual assistance in helping the victims of disease to overcome their problems. Documentary reports are now appearing, from medical centers as well as religious groups, that clearly establish the improvement of patients with strong religious beliefs. The recovery of such individuals is due to miraculous intervention according to them. Perhaps their faith allowed them to build up a strong immune system that eventually overcame their disease. All I know is that during my ordeal I had many men and women involved in church groups who offered me spiritual solace by their words and their prayers.

The miracles that are sought throughout the world are not always well received, but the prayers of the faithful are answered often enough to convince millions that there is a light at the end of the tunnel.

9
CROUP

Once A Deadly Disease

In the present era of antibiotics, there is almost total elimination of many diseases that were the scourge of the planet not too many years ago. For the present generation it must be hard to realize just over fifty years ago many common organisms like staphylococcus and streptococcus caused untold deaths and sometimes illnesses which left the patient incapacitated for months, even years, and sometimes for life.

As a youngster, I recall reading the news report of President Coolidge's son who died from a blister on his heel that became infected with the streptococcus bug. There wasn't any such thing as penicillin to treat the infection. One of the most devastating illnesses brought on mainly by the parainfluenza virus, but also a variety of other respiratory viruses, was croup which is basically laryngotracheobronchitis. This infection most commonly affected children under the age of six. The problem in croup is that it affects the airway passages, especially the larynx and the trachea, with variable involvement and spasm of the vocal cords. Since this is the gateway to the lungs, the swelling from the infection blocks off the breathing and if not relieved in time can cause death.

During my early years of practice an especially virulent form of croup occurred. It rapidly progressed down into the bronchi and lungs causing bronchiolitis or even pneumonia. This disease became almost epidemic. Treatment with penicillin was useless since it was caused by a virus. Early tracheotomy of such patients, often only two years of age or younger, gave some temporary improvement. However, within hours of surgery I would receive a call that the patient was having further difficulty. The inflammation which had started in the larynx had descended down the trachea and into the small bronchi. When the disease process reached the bronchioles, the smallest subdivisions of the bronchial tree were involved. The thick, tenacious mucus which developed could not be suctioned by the nurses' catheters through the tracheotomy opening.

In order to relieve the child's obstructed breathing, it was often necessary to take the patient to the operating room for bronchoscopic removal of the sticky secretions. By inserting this long metal tube through the tracheotomy opening, I could reach the mucus in the deeper part of the lungs. Some patients required bronchoscopy so often it became necessary to perform the procedure several times through the day and night. It was too exhausting for these small children to be carted back and forth to the operating room. It therefore became necessary to do the procedure at the patient's bedside. In spite of all these efforts, six of twelve affected patients failed to survive during an eight-week period in the winter of 1950.

At that time we had two children who were three and five years of age, a very troublesome age for childhood croup that year. I recall on several occasions when our youngsters developed a mild cough which usually occurred at night. Despite my wife's reassurance that they were "just coughing," I would frequently jump out of bed to check on them even if they just cleared their throats. Their mild spasmodic throat-clearing reminded me too much of the patient being seen in the emergency room because they could not breathe. These were the same type of children that sometimes required tracheotomy to keep their airways open and often failed to survive. Images like that floating in your brain weren't good for a restful night's sleep.

That period proved to be one of the most devastating in all my years of practice. The death of a child is always traumatic, but the almost complete helplessness in trying to overcome the effects of this tragic disease caused me many sleepless nights long after the epidemic had subsided. It was a year later that the "mycin" antibiotics were developed and the mixed organisms that produced this laryngotracheobronchitis were then brought under control. Over the years croup has become less of a threat to the well-being of children, but it still continues to be a serious disease that can be fatal.

Bacterial croup or epiglottitis must be differentiated from the viral croup that I have been discussing. This affects adults as well as children, but the smaller airway in youngsters contributes to a more frequent fatal obstruction of the breathing passages. The epiglottis acts somewhat like a trapdoor as it rests on top of the voice box and prevents food and liquid from going into the trachea and then down into the bronchial tubes and lungs. When it becomes swollen from infection the blockage to the airway may cause a fatality within hours if not recognized and treated properly. Because of the suddenness that occurs in crib deaths, the cause is often difficult to determine, but I believe that in some instances an autopsy might reveal inflammation and swelling of the epiglottis.

Epiglottitis is usually caused by Haemophilus influenzae type B.

During epidemics influenza type A virus is also a common cause of croup. The administration of antibiotics should control the symptoms and spread of epiglottitis, but the patient must be watched carefully. Any severe obstruction to the breathing may require immediate tracheotomy or the insertion of an endotracheal tube.

The suddenness and severity of this disease is no longer the threat it used to be, but its disastrous effects in the past cannot be easily forgotten by the parents and doctors who observed the fatal consequences in some of the children.

The Day I Cried

"I just had a call from the parents of one of my patients in Wethersfield. The child started to sound croupy a short time ago and now is much worse. They are on their way to the hospital now."

The 11 PM message from Dr. Desmond needed no further explanation. He was an excellent pediatrician and sensed that the patient was in extreme difficulty.

After alerting the emergency room, I contacted the operating room supervisor and alerted her to the possibility of a tracheotomy.

"I might not get back for a few hours since this sounds like a severe croup," I said to my wife. With these words I was out the door and headed for the hospital.

Three-year-old Christopher was carried into the emergency room within minutes of my arrival. His lips were blue and he had marked retraction of his chest and neck muscles due to his obstructed breathing. There was no time to ask for a detailed history since the diagnosis of croup was evident.

While Christopher was placed on the stretcher, the mother told me he had been fine all day.

"When he went to bed," she said, "he didn't even have a sniffle. But he woke up an hour ago sounding very croupy."

With the parents and emergency supervisor standing by, I immediately told them what had to be done.

"We are taking him to the operating room. He has to have an immediate tracheotomy to relieve the obstruction to his breathing."

Turning to the supervisor, I said, "The operating room was alerted about a possible tracheotomy before I left the house. Make sure the setup is ready with tubes for a three-year-old child."

There wasn't any time to discuss the procedure or the reason for the emergency with the parents, but as I dashed by I tried to reassure them that all would be well. I stayed by the stricken youngster's side as the stretcher was rolled toward the elevator.

Within moments after arriving at the operating room I had changed into an operating suit and was ready to make the incision.

To the anesthetist I said, "Place the patient on full oxygen and no general anesthesia. If you attempt to put him to sleep it could stop his breathing completely."

The operation went along uneventfully under local anesthesia. Moments after the tracheotomy tube was inserted the child's breathing became easier, his bluish color turned to pink, and I knew the immediate crisis was over.

To confirm the preoperative diagnosis, I inserted a laryngoscope into the boy's throat and examined the voice box area. As I expected, the epiglottis was a rosy red ball leaving only a tiny slit of an airway. It was a typical case of epiglottitis. Although Chris couldn't make any sounds because of the tracheotomy, his anxious look and gasping for air had disappeared. Each one of of us in the operating room began to smile with a great sense of relief. The tension of such procedures affects all of us who are involved and the joy is shared by everyone who has assisted in the operation.

After accompanying young Christopher back to the pediatric floor, he was immediately placed in a croup tent. This gave him a supply of oxygen and moisturized air during his convalescence for the next few days. The anxious parents were brought into the room where they were reassured of the operation's success.

"He still has his infection," I said, "but the tracheotomy will allow him to breathe without difficulty and in a few days the swelling should be reduced by the antibiotics."

That night I felt comfortable about the evening's events and slept peacefully. The following morning I checked Christopher before and after my operating schedule. He was breathing easily and the nurses reported that he had been experiencing no problems.

Several hours later, while I was in my office, a frantic call came from the pediatric nurse.

"Chris is having trouble breathing," she said, "and the suction catheter doesn't help."

Within a few minutes I was at the bedside and recognized the problem. The tracheotomy tube, which was very small because of the patient's age, had become obstructed with crusts. The nurse's suction catheter couldn't penetrate the blockage which had developed despite the moisturized croup tent. This had occurred in a few cases requiring that the tracheotomy tube be removed and a replacement inserted. Another similar tube was always kept in readiness at the bedside for such an emergency.

The replacement tracheotomy tube was checked and the portable light was set up to visualize the neck area. I removed the blocked tube with one hand and prepared to insert the new airway into the tiny tracheotomy incision. Suddenly a flash occurred and the light source went out. Apparently there was an exposed wire in the light cord and the moisture in the croup tent caused a short circuit.

As little Chris struggled for air I vainly tried to insert the fresh tube into the small opening of the trachea and reestablish the airway. Without a light source it was now impossible to find the tracheotomy incision which had become covered by the overlying edges of the skin.

Cradling Chris in my arm I told the nurses to call the OR and prepare a room for an emergency bronchoscopy. The elevator started moving upwards just as I reached its door. There was no way to get it back until its return from the top floor.

While dashing up the stairs for two floors to the operating suite, I continued to breathe frantically into the child's neck over the skin incision. My hopes were for the return of my little patient's color by bringing in some desperately needed air, but his lips remained blue.

Without waiting for gloves or gown, I ran into the operating room which had been readied for my patient. The lighted bronchoscope was inserted into the small but now easily visible tracheotomy incision. The anesthetist attached the oxygen which was forced in under pressure. Despite all our continuing efforts, Chris's color remained blue. His lungs remained completely collapsed and his heart had stopped beating. We couldn't revive him. It was one of the most shattering experiences of my life.

Leaving the operating room floor, I slowly walked downstairs to the pediatric section. There were few words to say to the parents except explain, as best I could, what had happened. Their grief was shared by me as I suffered the despair they experienced. Their only child seemingly rescued from death the night before was now taken away.

That evening I couldn't withhold my tears. In the practice of medicine we do have to restrain our emotions, but some events can be overwhelming. The death of Chris left me stunned and I couldn't control my feelings. He was the same age as my son, John. They both had red hair and freckles and this resemblance compounded my deep and poignant distress.

In reviewing the catastrophic events that had taken place, I realized that a precautionary measure could have been established. A suture thread inserted on each side of the incision would have readily exposed the area of the trachea. This would have allowed instant access to the surgical opening and prevented what developed into a disastrous fatality. I followed this precaution in subsequent tracheotomies, but no such mishap ever occurred again.

Allergies as a Cause of Croup-like Syndrome

An allergic reaction can precipitate a croup-like syndrome and if the cause isn't recognized and properly treated, a tracheotomy might be performed unnecessarily.

One morning I was asked to see the four-year-old son of a physician friend of mine. Their pediatrician had admitted little Johnny with a croupy cough several days earlier. Despite treatment and the continuous use of the croup tent, the patient's symptoms worsened.

The pediatrician, Dr Gaberman, asked me to evaluate the child with the thought of a possible tracheotomy. Johnny's breathing was becoming more difficult and his lips were noticeably blue, despite the use of the oxygen tent. He was definitely croupy, but he didn't have the usual history of a youngster with laryngotracheobronchitis. I also knew that the boy's mother had a severe sensitivity to cold air and cold water.

Since the croup tent was provided with cool moisturized oxygen, I suggested that Johnny be removed from the tent for several hours to observe his response. Within one hour he started to improve as his chest retractions and croupiness diminished. Two hours later his voice was almost normal. He was discharged from the hospital two day later.

The results were rather dramatic without resorting to surgery. It illustrated the importance of knowing a little bit of the family's personal background. Since I was a good friend and close neighbor of the parents, I was able to correlate the mother's sensitivities as a possible cause of her son's symptoms. I am sure that the mother's unusual response to a cold environment never gave her enough discomfort to inform the pediatrician of her problem.

Physical allergy, as it is called, has become universally recognized by allergists as a possible factor in producing croup-like symptoms in children and adults. However, in my early years of practice such a relationship wasn't too well known. Although it is now agreed that allergic responses can occur by exposure to heat, cold, and even exercise, the exact mechanism is not clearly understood. Again part of the treatment is the avoidance of exposure to the offending agent whenever possible.

10
DISEASES OF THE NOSE

Nasal Congestion

I saw a fifty-year-old man in consultation at the hospital because of nasal congestion which was present for many years. He stated he was able to obtain relief only with nose drops. My examination was essentially normal except for a marked deep-red congestion of his nasal membranes. It was a typical so-called "rhinitis medicamentosus," commonly known as "nose-drop nose," the condition that occurs from excessive use of nose drops. His sinus x-rays were normal.

"How often do you use nose drops?" I asked.

"About every three to four hours around the clock," he answered, "if I want to breathe properly."

"If you really want to clear up your congestion, you'll have to stop using the nose drops," I said.

He immediately reached down under his bed and dragged out a box containing a dozen bottles of Afrin which he pushed in front of me as he said, "OK, Doc, what am I going to do with all of these?"

It took a good while to convince this patient that Afrin was one of the worst offenders in causing severe nasal congestion and blockage when overused, as was certainly true in his case.

The patient had been originally admitted to the hospital for evaluation of vague stomach complaints which were traced to a mild gastritis. I ordered saline nasal douches which relieved his congestion. The saline douche is made with a pint of warm water and one teaspoon of table salt. This preparation works effectively in most cases of simple blockage. I also recommended that he continue these irrigations at home until he was completely normal and to avoid the use of Afrin. He called me two weeks later with the happy report that his nose was clear and that he was completely free of dependence on Afrin.

Alkalol, an over-the-counter preparation, has been used successfully by physicians for many years. I learned about this nasal astringent while attending a meeting in Boston. Dr. Lyman Richards, a member of the Eye and Ear staff gave glowing reports of its cleansing powers. Many of my patients who had become addicted to nose drops were able to kick the habit after conscientious use of Alkalol on a regular basis. One patient was advised by his druggist that it was the same as rubbing alcohol. The latter was used by this patient with disastrous results.

The Common Cold

This has to be considered the one infection that affects people more often than any other disorder. There are at least 200 different viruses associated with this disease. There is truly no such thing as a "common cold virus" and that makes the discovery of a cure well nigh impossible at this time. There are many contributing causes.

The sources of this nasal congestion are generally accepted as exposure to someone with the virus, low resistance because of fatigue, physical and mental stress, and of course allergies to inhalant substances including chemical irritants. Many allergic problems are diagnosed as simple colds until further investigation reveals that it may be may be an airborne allergen or even a food consumed by the patient.

The best treatment approach for the common cold is rest, if possible. The time-honored use of aspirin and forced fluids is most effective and the symptoms will usually subside in a few days.

Unfortunately, some patients feel that antibiotics should be started as soon as they get the sniffles. A call to the doctor often results in a prescription for an antibiotic to be used for three or four days. When the cold clears up as expected in that length of time, the cure is attributed to the medication. The cold sufferers who use this approach are hard to convince that such treatment builds up a resistance to the effects of the antibiotics. When a severe bacterial infection is encountered at some later date, the doctor and the patient are somewhat surprised to find there is no response to the antibiotic. Common colds shouldn't be treated this way unless the doctor sees evidence of secondary bacterial infection.

Nasal douching is often mentioned as part of the treatment in the relief of congestion of the nose commonly associated with colds, allergies, and the annoying postnasal drip. The solutions for clearing the nose can be enhanced by a modern and effective apparatus called the Water Pik. This simple gadget can reach the depths of the nasal passages more completely than the douche cup which has been a standby for so many years.

Allergy

The term allergy usually designates an abnormal reaction to a normal substance. It is generally agreed that this type of response affects at least ten per cent of the population. The exposure to chemical substances in the outside environment or in the confines of industry will also produce the added factor of an irritant that may cause symptoms similar to those caused by true allergies.

Seasonal allergies such as caused by trees, grasses, and weeds can vary in their intensity from mild bouts of congestion and sneezing to severe attacks of asthma. Perennial allergies are those occurring at any time during the year and a careful history is required to identify a specific allergen. Dust and animal dander are the most common offenders, but the problem of molds in the air, certain foods, and direct contact sensitivities can be a tremendous challenge to the physician in diagnosis and treatment.

Mild allergies can usually be controlled by over-the-counter medications that are now available. Any significant worsening of symptoms usually requires consultation with a physician. The allergist or the ENT specialist who includes allergy in his practice may suggest a series of skin tests to pinpoint the offending allergen.

Hypoallergenic pillows can give tremendous relief to those with a perennial nasal congestion. Most allergic patients are extremely sensitive to dust and their living areas should be thoroughly cleaned and protected against this source of discomfort. Air conditioning is recognized as an absolute must for any patient with allergic symptoms.

It is well established that animals carry a lot of dust in their coats. This, added to the natural danders found in cat and dogs and other animals, increases the sensitivity reactions of the patient. Keeping pets out of the sleeping areas and off the patient's lounging chair is most important. This is especially true during specific allergy seasons. Animal lovers are sometimes hard to convince that such steps are necessary.

Depending on the physician consulted and the variety of allergies, skin testing may involve up to several hundred or more skin pricks. This can be uncomfortable, tedious, and expensive. The RAST which is discussed in another chapter offers a simplified blood test that may prove to be just as effective in providing the information needed to make a diagnosis.

Food Allergies

"A man has just come in with difficulty breathing. He says that you are his physician."

The emergency room called me immediately and identified the patient as James Burke, a thirty-five-year-old patient who had been under my care for several years. This patient had been receiving injections for allergies to trees and grasses. He had been doing well, but it was noted, both by history and skin test that he was also allergic to molds as well as shell fish.

In the beginning he was advised to minimize his intake of his favorite beverage, beer. Foods such as oysters and shrimp had not caused any problems, but it was strongly suggested that he should avoid them during the allergy season.

On this warm summer day, he decided to stop off at the neighborhood tavern to quench his thirst with a glass of his favorite brew. He couldn't resist the tempting shrimp and oysters that were available at the bar. Within a short period of time he was on his way to the hospital with marked nasal and chest congestion.

His symptoms were quickly relieved by an injection of cortisone and after his allergic reaction there was no difficulty convincing him that beer and shell fish did not mix well.

Food allergies are becoming more widely acknowledged as a cause of nasal and pulmonary symptoms, sometimes extremely severe and life-threatening. The history is most important in tracing the connection between the food and the patient's problems. This is especially true of shellfish, peanuts, chocolate, and milk to name just a few of the common offenders.

Hidden substances in sauces, dressings, candies, and other mixtures have been determined to contain small amounts of allergens that have caused severe reactions and sometimes death. The food-sensitive individual has to be extremely careful about his or her intake and they must be constantly reminded of the deadly consequences if they dare to throw caution to the winds.

Nasal Polyps

Nasal polyps are grape-like growths found in one or both sides of the nasal passages. They are seen most often in allergic individuals and cause increased nasal blockage as well as sinusitis when complicated by infection. The occasional isolated polyp formation is easily controlled by surgical removal as an office procedure. Unfortunately, the polyps tend to multiply in very allergic individuals and that is when they invade the sinuses. Such an occurrence requires more extensive surgery, usually in a hospital setting. The laser is now found to be more effective in extirpating these growths when surgery is indicated.

The attempt to control polyps by injecting them with cortisone has not been too successful. The use of steroids by mouth or intramuscular injection will often reduce the size of the polyp and give the patient considerable relief, but this is only temporary. Although improvement is obtained from a nasal polypectomy, investigation for allergic and infectious causes is indicated to gain a more permanent relief of symptoms.

When sinus x-rays reveal clouding and probable infection of the sinuses, the likelihood of long-term help is difficult to predict. Sinus surgery can be successful and in many cases the patient will become symptom-free. The results aren't always predictable and it might be advisable to have a second opinion before deciding on extensive sinus surgery.

The Deviated Nasal Septum

The nasal septum is composed of bone and cartilage and is found in the midline of the nasal passages. Because of its location it commonly causes difficulty in breathing. In the past the problem was almost universally male-oriented. With the increased participation of women in contact sports we can expect a rise in the number of fractured noses and deviated septa among the so-called weaker sex.

Although the nasal bones give some protection to the septum, a blow to the nose can dislocate or bend this midline structure resulting in a blocked airway. Not infrequently, a blow to the nose may produce a hematoma (blood blister) on the septum. If not treated in time, an infection can result with loss of the cartilage and a decrease in support to the nose, causing a so-called saddle-nose deformity.

Any nasal trauma, especially in children, should be evaluated by the nose specialist for possible emergency treatment even in the absence of nasal fracture. Plastic repair of the septum with realignment of the nasal bones is often indicated if a good breathing result as well as cosmetic improvement is desired.

The moderate difficulty in breathing due to the deviation or displacement of the septum is often well tolerated by many sufferers. However, it may be the primary cause for recurrent attacks of sinusitis. The symptoms of moderate to severe headaches will develop in time because of the obstruction to the sinus drainage by the twisted septum. Septal surgery will allow the sinuses to clear their infected mucus more readily and often give the patient complete relief of his congestion and headaches.

Sinusitis

The ethmoid sinuses are groups of small cells located around the eye and are usually well-developed in childhood. When infected, the upper and lower areas around the eye as well as the face may become markedly swollen. Prior to the advent of antibiotics, surgical drainage was often necessary to diminish pressure on the eyeball and optic nerve which could produce blindness. Antibiotics now control most cases of ethmoiditis without resorting to surgery.

The frontal sinuses located above the eyebrows aren't well developed in childhood, but are commonly infected in adults and often accompanied by ethmoiditis. Most cases of acute frontal sinusitis are also treated successfully with antibiotics. When medication fails to control the infection, surgical drainage may be necessary to relieve the symptoms and also to prevent the more serious complication of brain abscess.

Sinusitis causing a severe toothache

Maxillary sinusitis may produce headache, although facial pain centered in the teeth area is often the first symptom of the disease. Usually this infection is mild and will respond to conservative treatment including antibiotics. The more severe involvement of the sinuses may cause extreme facial pain requiring immediate surgery to obtain relief.

John Pena was a good example of this. His wife called me and said, "My husband has a terrible toothache that woke him up early this morning. He saw his dentist who told him his teeth are fine and suggested that he see you immediately for his sinus."

John was a forty-two-year-old mechanic. When he developed his severe left-sided facial pain which became localized in his upper left molar he immediately sought relief from his family dentist. The pain was so severe, he admitted later, he insisted that the tooth be taken out. His dentist, however, recognized that the tooth was not infected and that the nerve roots in that area were inflamed by the pus and caused the pain. The dentist refused the patient's entreaties to remove the tooth and recommended ENT evaluation.

As expected, the x-rays showed complete clouding of the left maxillary sinus. Under local anesthesia, I inserted a long needle into the maxillary sinus and then injected warm saline solution under pressure. A large amount of foul-smelling pus was removed with immediate relief of the patient's pain. More importantly, the suspicion of a sinus infection by the family dentist also saved the patient the loss of a tooth.

11
NOSEBLEEDS

Treatment by the Patient

"Nosebleeds are the cause of more eye, ear, nose, and throat doctors becoming straight eye specialists than any other problems in the field of ENT."

This statement by the speaker at a seminar on nosebleeds had many approving nods of his listening audience, many of whom were continuing to practice E.N.T. as well as ophthalmology.

The combined specialty of eye, ear, nose, and throat was very common especially in the smaller communities. After many years of ear, nose, and throat practice I could readily appreciate why some physicians split their specialty and confined themselves to the clean and relatively bloodless eye diseases. They freed themselves of the frequent interruptions in their office schedule or their slumber at night when the urgent call was received from the patient with a nosebleed.

Most patients have learned that bilateral pressure on the lower nostrils, not the upper bony part of the nose, will stop the occasional dripping of blood. Such bleeding may occur from injury or blowing the nose too forcefully. Ice to the back of the neck, I do not believe, serves any useful purpose except to make the patient or the bystanders feel that something is being done.

When a patient rests the head back, the blood isn't seen because it's flowing into the back of the throat and into the stomach. For a short while the patient and the family feel more comfortable because no bleeding is noticed. However, any great amount of swallowed blood will eventually fill the stomach producing nausea and vomiting. The patient should be encouraged to keep the head forward while squeezing the nostrils to lessen the likelihood of accumulating blood in the stomach.

When there is heavy bleeding and clots fill the nasal passages, a firm blowing of the nose will expel the clots and help stop the blood flow.

Persistent bleeding can often be controlled by the insertion of cotton or paper tissue on the affected side. The use of a lubricating jelly,

131

which is preferable to vaseline, will minimize crusting and lessen the recurrence of mild bleeding.

Frequently recommended is the use of a vaporizer in the bedroom. This simple mechanical device is also aided by the placement of well-watered plants in the sleeping and living areas.

These are very effective ways of neutralizing the evaporating effects of our heating systems during the winter months.

A complete physical examination will help uncover hidden causes of recurrent bleeding related to medications and blood diseases such as leukemia and other dyscrasias.

Treatment by the Doctor

A family doctor referred a forty-eight-year-old man who had been experiencing mild nosebleeds intermittently for many weeks. The patient had several small bleeding points on both sides of the nasal septum. These areas were quickly controlled by electro-cauterization. The conjunctivae of his eyes were markedly pale indicating the blood loss was more severe than the history suggested. He was referred to the hospital hematologist who made a diagnosis of chronic lymphatic leukemia. Treatment was instituted and he was able to continue his work as an insurance executive for many years afterwards.

Simple cauterization of the bleeding vessel will often control the problem if the source can be seen in the anterior (front) part of the nasal septum. Heavy bleeding may require packing of the nose, sometimes on both sides.

Posterior nasal bleeding, common in adults, will require a gauze pack or a nasal balloon to be inserted into the back of the nose. Such a procedure should ordinarily be done by the ENT physician who has the experience and equipment to perform these approaches. As noted in an earlier chapter, posterior packing is uncomfortable for the patient and the physician. That first experience with a home visit convinced me that the family and the patient and the doctor are all happier when severe bleeding is controlled in the hospital environment.

For many years prior to and during my early period of practice the patient with excessive bleeding from the nose was packed and repacked. Multiple transfusions of blood did save lives, but on occasion some unfortunately died. When that happened everyone agreed nothing else could have been done.

It took some years and many deaths to convince a few doctors in major medical centers that some lives were being lost unnecessarily.

These intrepid researchers were able to devise approaches that would cut down the death rate as well as the period of hospitalization required to control severe bleeding from the nose.

Depending on the severity and source of the bleeding it was found there were several blood vessels that could be ligated to stop the flow of blood. It had been recognized that packing of the nose is successful in over 90% of the cases. However, if there was prolonged hospitalization and enforced bed rest because of continuous bleeding some complications and even fatalities were likely to occur.

A Grateful Patient and Son

"I would like to pay you for saving my mother's life."

Sophie's forty-year-old son was insistent on making payment and refused to wait until the billing at the end of the month.

The seventy-five-year-old patient had been experiencing nose bleeds that treatment by her family doctor failed to control. After being admitted to the hospital I saw her in consultation. The bleeding was definitely coming from the back of the nose and I inserted a posterior packing that temporarily stopped the blood flow. Despite transfusions and reinsertions of packs in the anterior and posterior aspects of the nose, some dripping of blood persisted.

On the third day of hospitalization the bleeding became profuse and I was called to see Sophie around midnight. All the packings were removed and after an intense search I located several bleeding points in the back of the nose which I cauterized. The nose was once again packed on both sides in the front as well as extra-heavy gauze rolls in the back. This controlled the bleeding although the packings were obviously quite uncomfortable.

It was some hours later, about 5 AM, when I received the call that my patient wasn't bleeding, but was having marked difficulty in breathing. Examination of this elderly lady revealed severe retraction of her chest and neck muscles as she was desperately pulling for air. Her lips had a bluish tinge and her throat showed no evidence of bleeding. However there was tremendous swelling of the soft tissues in the back of the throat. The patient's breathing was blocked off not only through the nose which was tightly packed, but also through the mouth. If the packings were removed, bleeding might recur. There was no question that an immediate airway had to be established by doing a tracheotomy.

Sophie was brought to the operating room where the surgery was quickly explained to her. I made the incision into the neck under local anesthesia, located the trachea, opened it, and inserted the tracheotomy tube. There was instant relief of the patient's breathing. Sophie reached out for my hand and drew it towards her lips. She couldn't speak because of the tracheotomy, but her lips moved in a silent "thank you" as she kissed my hand.

Later that morning, before starting my operative schedule, I met several members of the family, some of whom I hadn't met earlier when the tracheotomy was done. I explained why the surgery was necessary and also gave them the encouraging news their mother would make a full recovery.

That afternoon, while examining patients in the office, my secretary asked if I could spare a few moments to see Sophie's son. Despite talking to him earlier at the hospital, I thought he might need a few words of reassurance and suggested that he come into my consultation room. As he had done earlier that day, he thanked me effusively for the care given to his mother.

That's when he made the statement about wanting to pay me immediately for saving his mother's life.

I appreciated his kind words but protested any payment at this time.

"There's no need to pay now," I said. "We'll send the bill after your mother is discharged from the hospital."

However, this young man would not be dissuaded and insisted on making the payment. After figuring the time spent on packing the nose several times during her hospitalization as well as performing the tracheotomy, I asked the secretary to make out a bill for $200. The son reached into his pocket and counted out the amount from a roll of currency and departed with a happy smile on his face.

His mother completely recovered from her complicated nosebleed and I had the first of many experiences of caring for a Polish patient. I found patients of Polish descent not only grateful but always insistent on paying their bills promptly.

Sophie was one of many patients who were subjected to frequent nasal packings in my efforts to control nasal bleeding. Fortunately, the breathing difficulty she encountered didn't occur in other patients. It was some years later that artery ligation was devised which eliminated the need for prolonged nasal packing.

A Nosebleed and Death from Embolus

The call came from one of the busy internists on our staff.

"I've just admitted a sixty-year-old female with a severe nosebleed associated with high blood pressure. Would you please see her and do what's necessary to stop the bleeding?"

The patient was a very obese lady whose blood pressure continued to register well over 200 systolic despite her blood loss. Often the bleeding will produce a drop in the pressure which helps to stop the hemorrhage.

My examination revealed profuse bleeding from the left side of her nose, but no blood could be seen in the back of the throat. An anterior nasal pack was easily placed in the left nostril and the blood flow was easily brought under control.

Several days later, bleeding recurred and posterior packings were now required. Despite transfusions and bed rest the patient continued to bleed intermittently for three more days from both sides of the nose anteriorly and posteriorly.

I decided to place the patient under general anesthesia which would allow better visualization of the bleeding points in the nose. I cauterized the area and inserted new packing in the front and back of the nose. Further transfusions were given and in a few hours bleeding had completely stopped.

After forty-eight hours the packings were removed with no further evidence of bleeding. One week had now passed since the patient's admission and the family doctor agreed that recovery was sufficient to allow her out of bed. While walking toward the lavatory the patient suddenly collapsed and died.

The autopsy revealed an embolus in her lung. Limitation of her activities during the enforced bed rest, as well as her obesity and varicose veins, undoubtedly contributed to clot formation that traveled from the legs to the lungs.

Pulmonary embolus affects 500,000 people in this country each year with a 10% mortality. For many years most surgical patients were required to remain in bed for up to ten days following their operations. Death from a pulmonary embolus was common under these rules, but the reason wasn't clearly understood.

A Surgical Approach for Nosebleeds

A few weeks after the tragic death of the embolus patient, I attended a meeting in Chicago where one of the papers presented was on the surgical treatment of nosebleeds. The speaker was enthusiastic and positive as he explained his approach.

"I was discouraged," he said, "by the amount of time spent controlling nosebleeds and the occasional deaths that occurred despite my efforts. I knew that something had to be done."

This physician from St. Louis echoed my sentiments completely. He then described how he was able to achieve success.

"After tracing the branches of the carotid artery in the anatomy laboratory, I was able to determine the source of the bleeding exactly. By making a small incision on the side of the neck the correct branch of the carotid artery could be identified and ligated and the bleeding completely controlled."

This doctor's description of the surgical approach was so convincing I returned home and decided to use this method in my next case of persistent nasal bleeding.

Over a period of several weeks I spent Thursday, supposedly my free day, at the Yale Medical School anatomy laboratory. I carefully dissected and reviewed the neck tissues relating to the external carotid artery. In the 1950s very few ENT specialists had received training to prepare them for such surgery.

In subsequent months I had a number of patients where the bleeding had failed to be readily controlled by nasal packing. Without hesitation I told the referring physician why this type of surgery was indicated. The success in these patients resulted in an increasing number of consultations for surgical treatment of nosebleeds. The use of the artery ligation gave quick relief to the patients and the doctor. Frequent packings and repackings of the nose were no longer needed.

Although more than 95% of nosebleeds could be traced to a branch of the external carotid artery it was noted that despite nasal packings and even ligation some patients continued to bleed. Frequent transfusions as well as repeated packings of the nose were necessary before the bleeding subsided. On occasion some of these patients did not survive after ligation.

Research anatomists were able to trace the cause to the ethmoidal branch of the internal carotid artery. Tying off the branch from the external carotid wouldn't stop the flow of blood if it came from the ethmoid vessel. Ligation of the internal carotid artery itself wasn't feasible because that would affect vital structures in the brain. A safe approach for reaching and tying the ethmoidal branch was needed to stop the bleeding.

Learning this latest method was simplified by knowledge of the operating microscope and the acquisition of tiny surgical instruments necessary to perform this procedure. Again utilizing the facilities of the Yale Medical School anatomy laboratory I was able to perfect the technique required to reach this delicate area.

On some occasions the routine use of the external carotid artery branch ligation failed to stop the bleeding, as I mentioned previously. This required me to return the patient to the operating room and tie off the ethmoidal branch of the internal carotid. Eventually it became possible to properly identify the specific source of the bleeding.

The success in controlling nasal bleeding was a mixed blessing. To be recognized as having advanced knowledge in the treatment of nosebleeds was a satisfying feeling. However the calls for seeing these patients invariably, at least it seemed so, came during the evening meal or late at night. It was a reminder of the doctor's statement some years earlier:

"Nosebleeds are the cause of more eye, ear, nose, and throat physicians becoming straight eye specialists than any other problems in the field of ENT."

An Unexpected Request for Consultation

The call came to the office one afternoon from Sister Louise Pauline, a nurse supervisor.

"Come over right away," she said, "the patient is still bleeding."

"What patient?" I said.

"Dr. Victor's patient," she answered.

"Why are you calling me?" I asked.

"The patient was bleeding when he returned from the operating room so I called Dr. Victor. He told me to call Dr. Samuel who said he couldn't do anything and asked me to call Dr. Connolly. I called Dr. Victor again and told him Dr. Samuel couldn't take care of it and that he told me to call Dr. Connolly, but Dr. Connolly is out of town. Then Dr. Victor said to get anybody. Call Dr. Curran."

It was annoying to get this type of referral without even the courtesy of a personal call from the surgeon. I called the operating room and arranged for what I thought was the indicated surgery.

In any emergency you don't quibble about proper protocol. This had been an ongoing problem following the return of the younger surgeons from their years of military duty. The older doctors were in charge before the junior surgeons went off to service and they often failed to recognize or admit that the new breed had something to offer when they began practice.

The sequence of events leading to this referral actually started earlier that morning when the operating room supervisor asked me to delay a mastoidectomy that had been scheduled.

"Your scrub nurse is needed for a case in the room next door," she said in explanation.

"I don't mind waiting, but what is the emergency?" I said.

"Dr Victor has a patient with a bad nosebleed and he's going to tie off the carotid artery."

"Why the hell is Dr. Victor, a general surgeon, taking care of a nose-bleed?"

"The patient's ENT physician is Dr. Samuel," she said, "and he asked Dr. Victor to do the surgery."

Several members of our department had limited training and they preferred seeking consultation with some of the older surgeons who included nearly everything in their practice except brain surgery.

While waiting for my mastoid case to be started, I wandered into the room next door and watched the general surgeon at work. A young interne with an anatomy book opened to the diagram of the blood vessels in the neck, stood by Dr. Victor's side. He scanned the open page and the carotid artery branch was thus properly identified and ligated. No attempt was made to determine if the bleeding had been successfully controlled. My scrub nurse came back to the mastoid room and I did the mastoidectomy.

In the morning while I observed the operation by Dr. Victor on this patient, I knew that the branch of the external carotid artery had been correctly identified. However, the continued bleeding proved this artery wasn't the cause of the problem. Based on my previous experiences the source of the bleeding had to be the ethmoidal branch of the internal carotid.

Under microscopic vision, I made an opening between the nose and the eye until the back of the eyeball was exposed. I pushed the eye gently to one side, identified the ethmoidal artery, and blocked it off using a tiny metal clip. Inspection of the nasal area after removal of the packings showed no sign of active bleeding. I then closed the incision. The patient was discharged from my care several days later.

There was never any acknowledgement from Dr. Victor or Dr. Samuel that my efforts may have been instrumental in saving the patient's life. The failure to recognize another person's accomplishments isn't restricted to the medical field. However, it was somewhat distressing to encounter such a reaction when a patient's life is at stake.

Bleeding Controlled During Pregnancy

"This is Dr. Cohen and I have a twenty-six-year-old woman in her sixth month of pregnancy who has had nasal bleeding for over a week.

Her nose and throat doctor has been unable to stop the bleeding despite packing, transfusions, and artery ligations. Would you please see this patient and take care of her?"

This call from the patient's obstetrician came about 11 PM. I examined the patient and reviewed the history. She was a pleasant black woman with packs in both sides of her nose and incisions on each side of her neck.

Treatment in addition to the packings included transfusions totaling twenty pints of blood. A general surgeon had tied off the external carotid branch first on the left side and then on the right side with no improvement.

I decided after reviewing the history and examining the patient that the bleeding was coming from the left side and the left ethmoidal artery should be ligated. This was accomplished without difficulty shortly after midnight. The packings were removed and the patient was discharged four days later. Her obstetrician informed me she delivered a normal baby on her due date three months later.

The use of advanced surgical techniques which I found to be so successful were constant reminders that in the field of medicine the learning process never ceases. In fact it's absolutely necessary. Adopting these new procedures might be considered by others to be ego boosters, but each new bit of knowledge became an opportunity to make someone more comfortable or even save a life.

A Doctor's Son with Uncontrollable Bleeding

"Tim, this is Dave Gorman. I was called up here to see my son in a small town some sixty miles north of Bangor, Maine. Matthew, who is ten years old, has been attending a basketball camp for the month of July. This afternoon he got hit in the nose while he was playing and bled a lot from the left side of his nose. But then it stopped. He started bleeding again and they called me to say he had to be admitted to the only hospital in town."

"How is he doing now?" I asked.

"I arrived from Hartford an hour ago and he was doing OK, but in spite of the packing and a transfusion, the bleeding still continues off and on. What do you think?"

"Dave, it appears he has a serious problem and he might need a surgical ligation to stop that blood flow. There is no one whom I know in that area who can do the proper operation. It's now well after midnight and I would strongly recommend that you arrange for an ambulance to bring him down here to our hospital in Hartford."

"It may be some time before I can arrange for an ambulance and an attendant, but I should be able to get down to Hartford by 8 AM."

"Make sure that he is cross matched for enough blood and I will alert the operating supervisor to have a room ready for the surgery he will probably need."

It was 8 AM, just as I was ready to start my first operative case, when the call came from the emergency room that Matthew had been admitted. I hurried down to check on his condition. I saw a pale, apprehensive youngster with both sides of his nose packed with blood-tinged tampons. There wasn't any question that the history of his nasal bleeding indicated the necessity for a ligation of the ethmoidal artery.

After a quick greeting to the parents I accompanied the attendants as they guided Matthew to the operating room. As we moved off the elevator a sudden gush of blood came spewing out of Matthew's mouth. I knew immediately that the decision to risk the hazardous trip from Maine was correct.

Under endotracheal anesthesia the young patient was put to sleep and I made the curved incision between the nose and the eye. With the microscope in position I inserted a metal clip on the ethmoidal artery. I inspected the nose carefully after removing all packings and there was no bleeding.

Matthew was discharged from the hospital into the arms of his grateful parents several days later after his blood count had returned to normal. He had no ill effects from his bleeding or the surgery.

Injury to the nose rarely causes the severity of bleeding suffered by Matthew. However, when this does occur and continues it usually means that the ethmoid artery has been severed by a fragment of bone. When that happens the patient's blood loss can be fatal. Although I have seen this type of injury on several occasions during my years of practice, the circumstances in this case were most unusual. Since the parent was a physician and a close friend, there was an extra sense of responsibility in making the right decision.

The Source of Power to Stop Bleeding

A thirty-five-year-old male employee at a local chrome-plating company was referred by the company physician because of recurrent nosebleeds. After I examined him I inquired about the conditions at the factory.

"Are you expected to wear any protection against the fumes you say are there?"

"Yes, most of the time I wear a mask and there is a blower system to clear the air, but you can still feel the dryness in your nose."

My examination revealed crusts in both nostrils. I also found a small perforation in the septum which separates the nasal passages.

"Do you notice a whistling sound sometimes when you breathe through your nose?"

"Yes, I do, and my friends often ask me why I'm whistling. Is there a reason for it?"

I explained how the fumes at work cause the crusting which can eventually develop into a small hole. This can happen when the nose is picked to remove the crusts. The attempts at crust removal create the perforation by tearing off part of the mucosa of the septum along with the crust.

"Get some of this special lubricating jelly at the drugstore and use it twice a day. this will cut down the crusting and may help that hole to heal. Sometimes surgery is needed to patch up the opening, especially if you allow it to get big. However, don't forget to wear the mask at all times."

At the factory I found the blower system was being used to reduce the chromic acid fumes.

I suggested that it should be checked for its efficiency. Many of the workers weren't wearing their masks as required by company rules. The company physician was advised the mask rule should be strictly enforced. Most industries now realize if protective measures aren't being utilized the company is liable and that is costly.

After seeing a number of employees with the same nasal crusting and bleeding, I asked one worker if everybody had the same problem.

"Most of the men say they have noticed some nose bleeding, but one of the older guys was said to have the power to prevent this. I asked him where he got the power, but he wouldn't tell me."

"One more question," I said. "Will he give you the power?"

The answer came without hesitation.

"I asked him for the power and he said he could only give it to a woman."

Further questioning revealed the employee with the power was French and originally came from a small town in Quebec.

Several acquaintances of mine were of French parentage, but they couldn't enlighten me as to where I might find someone with the so-called power. I decided to check with the Franco-American Club located in the Frog Hollow section of Hartford. It was here that I was directed to an elderly gentleman who was aware of such mystical powers.

"Who do you know with that power?" I asked.

"My deceased uncle, who lived outside the city of Quebec, had the power. He had the power to stop bleeding and also to stop floods. I know all of these people were French, but none were women."

Like so much folklore, I was unable to track down any specific individual who had the power. However, all those with the secondhand information were convinced of the power broker's infallibility.

12
DISEASES OF THE EARS

Cleaning the Ears

"But doctor, how can I keep my ears clean unless I use a Q tip?"

This is a question often posed to the doctor. Unfortunately, many individuals feel they have to do something to help Mother Nature. Some believe they should take cathartics or enemas regularly. Others gargle with harsh antiseptics or without reason use nasal sprays.

Far too many are convinced they need vitamins in excessive amounts to ward off multiple diseases. A well-balanced diet supplies all the vitamins and mineral needed by the average person. If the patient insists they feel better taking vitamins then my advice is to take them. Some vitamins in excessive dosage, however, have been proven to cause problems.

It has been quoted for many years that "cleanliness is next to godliness," and so cleaning the ears becomes as much a ritual as brushing one's teeth, grooming the hair, or cleaning the fingernails. There is no question that a person, young or old, with a yellowish staining of wax on the outside of the ear canal is not the mark of a well-groomed child or adult.

In their attempts to achieve perfectly clean ears, many people resort to the well-known Q tip and in some cases even the blunt end of a hairpin. If they knew the anatomy of the ear they would be a lot more cautious and much less daring.

The outer ear canal is little more than a half-inch long from the outer edge to the drum. It's usually less than a quarter-inch wide. The wax that forms is normal and is considered to be a protection against contaminants to the drum. It also keeps the ear canal from becoming dry and cracking. The wax forms as tiny droplets which normally flow to the outer surface of the ear and disappear. They may stain the exit area of the canal and this is where the simple use of a face cloth prevents an unsightly appearance.

Any accumulation of wax deeper within the ear canal may eventually cause blockage of the hearing. Some individuals are more susceptible to this deposit than others, especially in the older age group.

Attempts to remove wax is approached in different ways by individuals and some of the ways are not recommended despite their popularity. It's a daily routine for many to let water run into the ears while taking a shower. Unfortunately, the water tends to swell up any accumulated wax, thereby causing increased blockage.

The more adventuresome believe that a Q tip is the method of choice and proceed to direct the cotton-tipped applicator into the canal. If the canal is narrow, any wax present will be pushed in deeper and often right against the drum. Immediate blockage or pain or both may then occur. If the ear canal is wide, the wax can be easily bypassed and the applicator will brush up against and sometimes penetrate through the drum with disastrous results.

Mothers have a tendency to clean the baby's ears with Q tips as a regular routine. This has been passed on from one generation to the next and any attempt to dissuade such methods is met with scorn.

In the practice of ENT there are many instances that can be recorded where little Johnny sees his mother do such a thing to his baby sister and then tries the same thing on his own ears. Not infrequently this results in a bleeding ear and sometimes perforation of the drum.

It's not uncommon to be asked to examine a youngster with a piece of cotton embedded deep in the ear canal left there by the mother's use of the Q tip. Very often this is noted by the pediatrician during a routine examination. Sometimes because of its deep location and lack of proper instrumentation, the child is referred to the ear physician for safe removal of this foreign body.

There are a number of preparations on the market which are effective in breaking up wax accumulation. I have found that products such as Cerumenex and Debrox work quite well. Some physicians prefer mineral oil as a softener. The use of softeners followed by a gentle irrigation of warm water may avoid a visit to the doctor.

In some individuals there may be a sensitivity to over-the-counter ear-softener preparations which can cause irritation of the lining of the ear canal. In such cases their use should be discontinued and the patient should be seen by the physician. Occasionally the wax may be impacted in the ear canal and doesn't respond to gentle irrigation by the parent. A visit to the doctor is most important since vigorous attempts to remove the wax can be harmful.

To avoid trouble it might be advisable to remember an age-old admonition: "Never put anything into your ear smaller than your elbow wrapped up in your overcoat."

Earache — A Midnight Family Emergency

Acute infection of the middle ear has always been a very common problem of children and produces pain with some hearing loss. Treatment of the acute infection with antibiotics and pain medication will usually be successful with complete response in several days. Prior to the advent of antibiotics, the only relief that could be obtained was by myringotomy (incision of the drum). This gave instant relief of the pain and certainly helped reduce the incidence of acute mastoiditis, a dreaded disease before 1950.

Our three-year-old son, John, awoke at midnight with intense ear pain that failed to respond to medication. His screams sent shock waves of discomfort through my wife and me. Timothy, his five-year-old brother lying next to him, covered his ears trying to block out the sounds of John's piercing wails.

Examination with the otoscope revealed an ear drum that was bulging and fiery red. If myringotomy wasn't done the pain would undoubtedly continue for many hours until the force of the pus ruptured the drum. Calling one of my ear colleagues and bringing John to the hospital for anesthesia and surgery would prolong his discomfort for several more hours. There was also the added hazard of the general anesthetic, ether, which was safe but not without some danger.

My wife and I finally decided that immediate home surgery was the fastest and the best solution. With Mary's nursing skill, John was securely wrapped in a sheet while I set up my head mirror and light. The ear speculum was inserted, the swollen drum visualized and quickly pierced with the myringotomy knife. There was an instant outburst of screeching pain from John who then lay back quietly and within seconds went to sleep. He had no further difficulty that night or in the years afterwards.

His brother burst into tears when John emitted his loudest scream as the myringotomy was done. The sobbing Timothy was comforted by his mother and soon dozed off to join John in slumberland.

It was a difficult decision to make that night, but I knew there was no other way to relieve John's discomfort quickly and avoid any possible complications. Antibiotics have long since eliminated the need for such an emergency surgical procedure.

Serous Otitis Media

This fluid condition, most common in children, produces hearing loss of varying degree, but is not accompanied by pain or fever. Although mastoiditis is rarely encountered in the present day, the advent of antibiotics may have paved the way for the development of this middle ear fluid which often occurs after the acute ear infection has subsided. In some cases the fluid formation appears related to allergies or enlarged adenoids.

Hearing loss, which develops from serous fluid, is not always recognized by the parent since it may be gradual rather than instant. Typically, the child who has been a good student falls behind in his studies, but quickly develops the ability to lip-read. He is often considered inattentive since he seems to hear "what he wants to hear." Routine hearing tests in school will frequently help to pinpoint the problem.

Treatment of this type of hearing loss has undergone some changes depending on the physician consulted. Immediate myringotomy with insertion of a small plastic tube to prevent the reaccumulation of the fluid is the approach of some ENT specialists. Other doctors recommend continuance of decongestants and antibiotics for long periods of time despite the failure of the child's hearing to improve.

Incision of the drum along with insertion of the drainage tube usually gives instant return of hearing. Although this seems to be the preferred approach in most cases, many physicians including some otologists, now recommend a trial of conservative treatment before any surgery. With a little patience on the part of the parent and the doctor, the problem might be resolved without an operation, but extensive delay is not in the best interests of the child.

"Glue ear" is a type of serous otitis that is usually present for a long period of time and myringotomy cannot be avoided. Insertion of a large-bore plastic tube which remains in place for many weeks or months may be necessary until the disease process clears. In some cases the "glue ear" invades the mastoid and a simple mastoidectomy may be required.

A Self-inflicted Injury

The office schedule was interrupted one morning by the visit of a thirty-year-old male, George O'Neil, who was holding a blood-tinged handkerchief to his ear and complaining of pain.He quickly recounted the history which he had given to the secretary as I prepared to examine the ear.

"Well, Doc," he said, "I was cleaning my ears with a Q tip just before leaving for work, but my wife started to nag me about putting those things in my ear. I told her that I had been doing that for years and it helps to keep my ears clean.

"She kept yakking away about how dangerous it was. She had read something in one of those women's magazines about all the things that can happen. Well, finally I got mad and left the table and rushed toward the doorway.

"That's when she yelled out, 'You've got that Q tip in your ear.'"

"'I know I have it in my ear,' I told her, as I slammed the door and that's when it happened. The door hit the Q tip and I thought I would go through the roof with the pain. I put my hand to my ear and it was covered with blood. Then I noticed I couldn't hear and that really scared me. Tell me, Doc, will I be all right?"

"I can tell better in a few minutes," I said, "but first let me take a look."

The outer ear was covered with blood and the ear canal itself was clogged with it. This took some time to clear away before I could see the bleeding points in the canal. Cauterization quickly controlled the bloody discharge and allowed me to visualize the drum which had a large central perforation where the Q tip had penetrated.

A quick whispered-voice test indicated that the hearing was essentially normal and George was reassured that his injury had not affected the hearing bones. He was also advised that the slight diminution of hearing which was present would clear up as soon as the drum healed completely as anticipated. Whenever the hearing bones are fractured or dislocated by any trauma the sound reception is diminished by as much as 50% and would require major reparative surgery.

The edges of the broken drum were gently laid back in place where they became approximated. No patch was indicated at this time.

A large cotton ball was now placed in the outer canal for protective purposes and the patient was given a prescription for an oral antibiotic. He was cautioned against getting water or any other ingredients into the ear canal.

The patient was seen at one week intervals for three weeks. By that time the drum had completely healed and his hearing was within normal limits.

Nature often has a way of healing many drum injuries without the doctor having to resort to surgical attempts at closure. If a perforation has been present for a long period of time, it indicates that nature's healing process has not occurred because of the extent of the injury or the added complication of infection.

Some drum perforations may require immediate application of a cigarette paper or, as one otologist suggested, a piece of condom. This type of patch is needed if the drum edges cannot be approximated. The more resistant cases may need a skin or muscle graft to assure success. In addition, as noted earlier, the break in the bony chain demands more advanced procedures to restore the continuity of the sound mechanism. The development of the operating microscope has been a real boon to the ear physician in improving the results for restoration of hearing.

When Nature Heals the Ear Drum

The patient was Bill Curley, a nineteen-year-old college student who was not uncomfortable, but concerned that after swimming and occasionally showering, his left ear would drain.

"When did all this start?" I asked.

"It began about three months ago after wrestling with my roommate at school. His hand accidentally hit me in the left ear and it started to ring. Then I noticed that I could hear, but not as clearly as on the right side. The school doctor gave me some ear drops which stopped the discharge. Lately there hasn't been any drainage, but the sounds on the left seem muffled. What did my test show?"

"The hearing test by my audiologist shows a slight loss," I said, "but let's see what the drum looks like."

A quick examination of the ear revealed the problem.

"You have a good-sized hole in the middle of your eardrum. There is no infection present, but whenever water gets into the canal, especially from swimming, it may set up the discharge and increase the hearing loss."

"How can the drum be healed?"

"In your case, since the eardrum is dry, it may be possible to close the perforation with a simple graft which I can apply here in the office. If that doesn't take, then it may be necessary to admit you to the hospital for a muscle or skin graft."

After properly preparing the drum edges, a cigarette paper patch was applied over the perforation. The patient was advised to cover the ear while showering and to do no swimming. He was returning to school in a few days for the fall semester and an appointment was made to have the ear examined again when he came home for the holiday vacation.

The checkup in December showed no sign of the patch which had completely disappeared as occasionally happens. The perforation was still present with no apparent change in size.

I now made my next recommendation.

"You are going to require a muscle or skin graft to close that opening, otherwise you risk developing infections every time you get any water in your ear. That surgery will be done when you return home for the summer vacation."

"I've signed up for a summer job when school closes. Could you do the operation as soon as I return home?"

"After all these months with no change in the perforation there is little likelihood that the drum will heal over. We will arrange for your admission to the hospital the day you return home and the operation will be done the next morning. If the ear has any drainage or causes any discomfort at the time of admission make sure you call my office. The surgery won't be done if there is any infection."

Unfortunately, Bill was delayed in returning home from school and it was late in the evening when a call was finally received that he was admitted to the hospital. I talked to him on the phone and he assured me that the ear wasn't draining and he was looking forward to the operation the next day.

After greeting my patient in the operating room the next morning, I went to the scrub area and then gowned myself for the surgery. The microscope was wheeled in place and I now looked into the canal to prepare the area for the grafting procedure.

What a surprise! The drum perforation was completely healed over and the rough whispered test indicated essentially normal hearing.

"Bill," I said, "I have good news for you. Your drum is completely healed and there is absolutely no sign of the hole that had been there three months ago. I am discharging you today and want to see you in the office tomorrow when I'll do a more complete hearing test. As of now I would say that you are cured."

There was no explanation as to why an unhealed perforation completely closed over despite the failure to show any activity toward healing during the first three-month period. The waiting interval in this case was successful, but I would hesitate to suggest this as an approach in every case.

Hearing evaluation the following day showed a normal response and my patient was advised that he could engage in his usual activities. I did suggest that diving might cause a problem since the healed drum was thinner than normal tissue and might not withstand the pressures of deep diving.

Bill was reexamined twice in the succeeding months and healing remained complete. Nature has a way of healing many kinds of injuries, but the repair of this large drum perforation gave me much food for thought. There is an old saying oft repeated, "You can't fool Mother Nature." This time Mother Nature fooled me.

Sudden Loss of Hearing and an Unusual Cure

The fifty-five-year-old male patient, George Mooney, presented himself with a history of hearing loss which was frightening because of its suddenness and severity.

"I don't know what happened to my hearing, Doctor. I was doing some paper work in my office and the left ear became completely blocked. It started off with some ringing and within seconds I couldn't hear a thing from that side."

"Did you get hit in the ear accidentally or otherwise?" I asked. "Were you dizzy or exposed to any loud noises nearby?"

The answers to all these questions were in the negative.

Examination of the ear canal showed no wax and the drum appeared normal. Tuning fork testing was done and indicated a severe loss of bone conduction which meant that the hearing nerve was affected.

"Let's get some more hearing tests from the audiologist and that might give us a clue as to what the problem is and what we can do to help."

The complete audiological results confirmed that the patient had a severe loss affecting the hearing nerve and not the hearing bones. The history of this type of hearing loss is reported as not being too common and the cause is not easily identified.

Some otologists have suggested that the round window in the middle ear has ruptured, but this has not been fully authenticated. Another theory is that an embolus (blood clot) has blocked off a small blood vessel in the inner ear. Other investigators have pushed the idea of a virus which is a common guilty culprit for many diseases when we can't find a reason that can be identified.

On the basis of the cause being a possible blocked blood vessel, I placed the patient on a vasodilator drug called nicotinic acid. This has been used by several otologists who published encouraging results. I also told him to go to bed early and get a good night's rest. I didn't try to be too optimistic since the outlook really wasn't favorable.

"Call me in the morning and we can decide what else we might try if you're no better."

The next morning he gave me his report.

"Doctor, I took the two tablets as you suggested," he said, "and when I woke up this morning I could hear fine."

"That's great, George," I said, "because the treatments for this kind of problem are limited and there is no guarantee of cure with anything we might do."

"One other thing, Doc," he said, lowering his voice as if he was going to reveal a deep dark secret. "Do you think it was the medicine or the two shots of V.O. whiskey that I took with the tablets?"

Although alcohol is considered a vasodilator, I decided to label the treatment and the report as anecdotal rather than a suggested cure. I never saw a patient with a similar history so I had no occasion to use the same type of treatment on another individual with sudden hearing loss.

The Hucksters Selling Hearing Aids

Difficulty in hearing can be devastating to the individual depending on the amount of loss and his occupation. Again, a lot depends on the patient's acceptance of his deafness. In some cases of severe nerve deafness, I've found that despite the best of evaluations and advanced treatments the chance of improvement with a hearing aid may be minimal. This is especially true in patients who are victims of Meniere's disease in which there is marked loss of discrimination with the ability to hear but not understand what is said.

After my explanations and counseling, I've been somewhat disturbed to find that very frequently some patients have responded to a TV commercial, a newspaper ad, or a telephone call for a home evaluation of their hearing loss. A smooth-speaking sales person convinces them his highly-advertised aid is a new breakthrough. The gullible patient, often a most intelligent and questioning person, signs on the dotted line for a hearing aid costing twice as much as instruments sold by reputable dealers.

In practically every instance the victims later turn to me, crestfallen and embarrassed, as they admit they were taken. It should be emphasized that any individuals, especially those with a severe hearing loss, should be evaluated by a physician who is a recognized specialist in ear diseases. The specialist can determine if the deafness is a life-threatening problem or one that is treatable by medicine, surgery, or the use of a hearing aid.

Those physicians seeing patients with hearing problems become concerned when they encounter more and more victims of unscrupulous hearing-aid dealers. The officers of our state ENT society asked that I meet with a representative of the dealers and work out an acceptable agreement. Nothing could be accomplished until it became necessary to mandate an enforceable law.

It was finally decided that no hearing aid could be sold without a written agreement that the patient had sixty days to return it if dissatisfied. It was also required that no aid could be sold without a stipulation of approval from a physician, preferably an ear, nose, and throat doctor.

The latter restriction was often overcome when the dealer prompted the clients to sign an affidavit that they did not wish to see a doctor for an extra-charge visit. The new regulation was not foolproof, but it did inhibit the dishonest dealers from taking advantage of many unsuspecting individuals.

Treatment with Acupuncture

The mother of a twelve-year-old youngster brought the severely deafened child to my office for evaluation. The prime purpose of the visit was for me to give an opinion regarding the value of acupuncture in the treatment of deafness. This was being promoted by a physician in the city of Springfield thirty miles away.

From my earliest years of practice I found that the young patient and his family should never be told that "nothing can be done" for any problem at hand. They must always be encouraged to search for the "light at the end of the tunnel" and never give up hope. However, in the meantime, they must be advised to use the facilities available such as the school for the deaf which this young man attended.

My examination including audiometric testing revealed profound hearing loss. When it came to making a recommendation for acupuncture, I told them there was no scientific evidence that this type of treatment for deafness was beneficial in any way.

At this point the mother stated she had already made an appointment and was quite determined to have the course of four treatments. Each visit was to cost $35.00 and the course of acupuncture applications would take place over a period of one month. The average specialist charge for an ear exam in Hartford at this time was $5.00. As could be readily seen, the acupuncture cost was exceptionally high.

I told the mother that I would be happy to see her son again at no charge at the end of his treatments and strongly suggested she shouldn't have her hopes set too high.

In a month's time she returned with her son and proudly announced that the tests by the acupuncture specialist showed a definite improvement in his hearing. After my examination and hearing test I showed the mother the results and compared the findings with my previous evaluation. There was absolutely no change in the youngster's hearing.

The mother then agreed she herself hadn't noticed any improvement in her child. She finally realized that further acupuncture treatments, which had been advised, would be futile.

She decided to continue with his program at the school for the deaf and accept for the present at least that there was no treatment except the use of a powerful hearing aid, lipreading, and auditory training.

Dizziness and Facial Paralysis

Cholesteatoma is a benign tumor that develops from a chronic middle ear infection that extends into the mastoid. This growth eventually may cause deafness as well as dizziness, facial paralysis, and sometimes brain abscess. Mastoidectomy is absolutely indicated to relieve the problem and prevent further complications.

Stanley was a forty-eight-year-old patient of Polish birth who gave a history of dizziness for many months. His intermittent attacks were not severe and his family doctor prescribed medications that seemed to help. The dizziness wasn't incapacitating, but continued to recur and the attacks were often accompanied by nausea.

One morning Stanley awakened and noticed that his face was twisted. This upset the patient and his wife considerably. I had seen her previously for a sinus infection and at her suggestion he agreed to an evaluation by me.

Examination revealed a definite facial paralysis on the left side. The ear canal showed only a minimal amount of secretion, but I suspected a mastoid infection when the cotton swab used to wipe the area had a definite foul odor. The patient at first denied knowledge of any ear discharge, but then he recalled having been subject to ear infections many years earlier when he lived in Poland.

After thoroughly cleaning the ear canal and viewing the drum through the microscope, I was able to see a pinpoint opening high up in the drum. It was almost obscured by the ear canal wall. My suspicions of a cholesteatoma were immediately aroused and the possibility of this dangerous condition was explained to the patient and his wife.

The x-rays of the mastoids by the radiologist confirmed the diagnosis. The films revealed a huge cholesteatoma that must have been growing for many years. Surprisingly, there was very little loss of hearing. The auditory ossicles had escaped any involvement with this insidious growth and in view of its large size this was most unusual.

I had the patient admitted to the hospital immediately and performed mastoid surgery on him the next day.

The bone covering the facial canal was eroded by this nonmalignant, but very invasive growth that was pressing on the facial nerve and causing the paralysis. The adjacent bone of the equilibrium canal was also affected by the cholesteatoma and this was the cause of his recurrent dizziness. As noted in my office examination, Stanley's hearing was within normal limits and at surgery the auditory ossicles were completely intact with no involvement by the invasive mass.

Recovery from the dizziness and the paralysis took almost a month, but at the end of that time, Stanley could smile normally and walk without any unsteadiness. Cholesteatomas, such as experienced by this patient, are usually identified by the early examination of the ENT physician. Usually, hearing loss has developed because the auditory ossicles are involved in the infectious process. The onset of dizziness is also commonly associated with the development of this growth. There are so many cases of unsteadiness among patients that frequently a long delay in the diagnosis occurs while the patient may be treated as Meniere's disease or something else.

Brain Abscess and Aphasia

"Would you see a patient of mine who has a draining left ear and the x-rays show a cholesteatoma on that same side?"

The request came from one of the ENT physicians who didn't perform mastoid surgery. This referral proved to be a most interesting and somewhat unusual case. The patient was a forty-two-year-old man, Vincent, who had a discharge from his ear for several months without any other symptoms. The diagnosis of cholesteatoma prompted his doctor to seek another opinion.

After I examined the films I saw the patient in the microscope room. In addition to the drainage in the left ear there was a large perforation of the drum on its upper edge. My suspicion of involvement beyond the ear occurred when routine questioning revealed the patient's inability to identify common objects such as a key or a pencil.

I held up a pencil and asked, "What is this, Vincent?"

After a few moments, looking puzzled, he replied, "I can't remember."

"Is it a key'"'

"No."

"Is it a knife?"

"No."

"Is it a pencil?"

"Yes."

There was no doubt that the cholesteatoma had invaded the brain causing a symptom known as amnesic aphasia. I requested a consultation from a neurosurgeon who agreed that a combined ear and brain approach was indicated. I opened up the mastoid and removed the large cholesteatoma and the neurosurgeon cleaned out the subdural area where the growth had invaded the brain.

The neurosurgeon and I examined the patient daily after the operation. He was healing nicely.

By the third day I held up a key and asked, "What is this?"

The patient had a smile on his face as he responded, "A key."

Several other objects were also identified correctly. We knew that the operation was a success. The patient made an uneventful recovery and was discharged from the hospital one week later.

13
HEARING LOSS

In Search of a Cure for Deafness

"Doctor, I can hear!"

These are the most comforting words for the patient to express and the doctor to receive when the person with a hearing loss has undergone a successful surgical procedure.

In the early 1900s, and years before that, there were many attempts to treat patients with a hearing loss. The ear specialists from the most prestigious medical centers advised their patients and fellow physicians about the newest vitamins that were available to bring new hope to the deaf.

The blowing of air into the nose causing increased pressure on the ear drum gave some patients instant improvement in hearing loss related to a recent upper respiratory infection. This induced many physicians to use the same treatment on long-standing hearing loss that was often related to nerve deafness. The patients were often advised that the treatments must be continued weekly for many months to gain improvement which, of course, never occurred. The attempts were doomed to failure.

A monthly magazine called Mercury, published a widely-circulated article on hearing loss in early 1950, "New York Specialist Discovers Cure For Deafness." This highly-publicized article was given much attention in the press and on radio. It was a complete hoax pushed by an osteopathic physician with an office on Park Avenue.

By inserting his finger into the patient's mouth, he massaged the tissues in back of the nose. He claimed the restoration of normal hearing in hundreds of deafened individuals and even hired a writer to have the article published.

In rare instances some blockage of the eustachian tube might be cleared by this maneuver and possibly give the patient a temporary improvement. Two patients that I saw in my office confessed they had taken the long trip to New York and paid the fee of $500.00 in advance for the series of treatments. There was no further charge, but like all the others, the patients I saw had received no improvement. After many trips to the Big Apple for their weekly massages, these two patients became disenchanted and finally stopped the treatments.

In 1890, Dr. Frederick Jack, a surgeon at the Massachusetts Eye and Ear Hospital was able to restore hearing in several patients by removing one of the auditory ossicles, the stapes. Unfortunately, there were complications such as meningitis and often death following the procedure. Without the benefit of magnification and microscopic instrumentation and no protection from antibiotics, Dr. Jack finally gave up what was initially a successful operation. There were no further attempts by other physicians to emulate his pioneering surgical procedure.

A Nonsurgical Approach to Deafness

A new approach in controlling otosclerosis has been the use of sodium fluoride. When taken by mouth on a daily basis, the researchers who have followed patients for two or more years claim that during this period the patients' otosclerosis had been prevented from progressing. It's important to see the patient before the deafness has reached a point where there's difficulty in communication. The medication doesn't loosen the fixation of the stapes that causes the hearing loss. That can only be done by surgery.

By diagnosing patients in the early stages of otosclerosis, usually their hearing will not be impaired by the time treatment is begun. With an 80-85% success rate in patients on the fluoride capsules there is a great deal of enthusiasm on the part of the physicians who are using this treatment.

For those who have already developed a hearing loss which impairs their ability to understand what is being said, the use of a hearing aid or surgery offers the best chance to cope with the problem. The technological advances in the construction of hearing aids have allowed millions of deafened men, women, and children to join the hearing world once again.

Cochlear implants when first developed required a huge box-like accessory to allow sound to be brought to the profoundly-deafened patient. Miniaturization of the components has made it possible for such individuals to wear all the equipment needed and with the help of trained speech therapists they are able to carry on reasonable conversation. Although this present system of communication leaves much to be desired, the world of complete silence has now been opened again for many. In some cases they are hearing and understanding words for the first time. I believe cochlear implants offer a real hope for the patient who was faced with an uncorrectable problem.

Many individuals are able to minimize their difficulties by lipreading. This requires exact attentiveness on the part of the hearing-impaired. Also, the speaker is sometimes embarrassed by the intensity of the listeners watching his lips.

There is just no easy solution for the hearing-impaired, especially for the individual who develops a severe hearing loss late in life.

The Fenestration Operation

A better understanding of the disease process called otosclerosis occurred in the 1940s. This disorder causes the stapes hearing ossicle to become fixed and prevents sound waves to be transmitted to the inner ear. It was at that time a New York ENT physician, Julius Lempert, devised the fenestration operation. This six-hour procedure was approached very cautiously by the older ear physicians whose past experience with surgery for deafness had been unsuccessful.

A number of younger otologists studied under Lempert and learned the new technique. They reported their results with the same successful rates as claimed by Lempert. It was the first major breakthrough in the successful treatment of otosclerosis and now became accepted by a number of ear surgeons. After visiting Lempert's hospital and watching him operate I was impressed with his surgical technique. The results reported by Lempert as well as the doctors who studied under him were impressive.

The course offered was given twice a year at his hospital in New York and was limited to four board-certified ENT specialists. I felt fortunate in being accepted for the midwinter session which lasted six weeks. During that period it was necessary to close my office for any patient care. The training program was an all-day affair for five days each week. I found a hotel close to the hospital where the room rates were cheap. It was called the Princess, but it was a real fleabag, certainly not the place where royalty ever stayed.

At the small hospital owned by Lempert, skulls were supplied for dissection in a laboratory. The students were given all the equipment necessary to perform the fenestration operation. In the morning we observed the surgery performed by the master himself, Dr. Lempert, or one of his two associates. The afternoon was devoted to the laboratory dissection and the evening sessions were supervised by Dr. Dorothy

Wolf, a pathologist. She explained how otosclerosis developed and why it caused deafness. She was a meek little woman who almost seemed to cringe when Dr. Lempert would on rare occasions let loose with a string of expletives during an angry moment.

The charge for the course was $1800. My hotel room cost $100 a week and, of course, it was necessary to maintain my office staff of a nurse and secretary at full wages. In those years the office fees had been established at $5.00 and tonsillectomy patients were charged $25.00. The few years that I had been in practice gave me an opportunity to develop a strong following of patients. There wasn't too much of a nest egg to dig into, but despite the financial sacrifice I was determined to learn the newest approach to combat deafness.

After completing the fenestration course, I now reviewed the cases of otosclerosis that were maintained in my files. During the subsequent few months several of these patients were offered the operation as an opportunity to regain some of their hearing.

The fenestration could not restore speech reception to normal, but it could possibly eliminate the need for the hearing aid that many were using. In the beginning the early results were encouraging and the operation was performed on a dozen patients.

In performing fenestration surgery it is necessary to do a mastoidectomy. Despite improved hearing initially, some patients developed ear drainage. Later these patients began to lose their hearing. The surgery didn't worsen the patient's hearing, but I felt there had to be a better way to help the deafened.

The training I received by Lempert and his associates gave me an expanded knowledge in the anatomy and control of many diverse ear infections. The use of magnification, the electric drill, and other new instruments allowed me to clear ears of infection that had defied the efforts of surgeons prior to that time.

Stapes Mobilization

"You are nothing but a charlatan trying to foist a bad operation on all these doctors."

This shocking statement by Dr. Julius Lempert caused a buzzing of excitement at the ENT meeting held in Atlantic City.

His remarks were aimed at Dr. Sam Rosen who had described his success in obtaining normal hearing in patients with otosclerosis. He called the procedure "stapes mobilization" and it seemed reasonable and simple to perform. The stapes bone is shaped like a stirrup. the footplate of the stapes is the portion of the bone that becomes fixed, thus preventing the transmission of sound. Rosen wiggled the footplate loose with a simple maneuver allowing the stapes to move freely once again and pass the sound waves to the inner ear.

Dr. Rosen, a mild-speaking man, tried to convince Lempert that his operation was successful.

"Julius," he said, "you should try this procedure yourself and see how well it works."

"Before doing my fenestration," Julius replied, "I had mobilized the stapes and it didn't help the hearing."

For some minutes bedlam ensued as the supporters of fenestration stood up en masse and defended their procedure. When it all quieted down I was in a state of confusion as were many others who watched and listened to the arguments.

The stapes operation was simple and could be performed in a half hour or less. No mastoidectomy was required as with the fenestration and the results were immediately apparent when the surgery was completed. Hearing loss in otosclerosis occurs, as I mentioned before, when the footplate of the stapes becomes fixed by bony growth. The sound waves are no longer transmitted and the patient's hearing loss develops. Cracking that tiny footplate allows movement of the ossicle and sound waves can once again be heard.

Unfortunately, as with any fracture in the body, the break in the bone heals. The stapes footplate becomes refixed after several months. Despite good results initially in seven of my ten cases, I decided to seek a better way of assuring my patients of more permanent hearing improvement.

Stapedectomy

"What is your assessment of John Shea?"

This question was directed by Dr. Brown Farrior of Tampa to friends of his who supervised the training of residents at the Massachusetts Eye and Ear Infirmary in Boston.

"He is a fine young man, but he doesn't do things our way," was their answer.

"When I heard their answer," Dr. Farrior said, "I decided that Dr. Shea had a bright future. I'd rather see a man fall flat on his face going forward than fall on his ass leaning backwards."

Dr. Farrior was a well-established otologist who conducted a course in ear surgery at St. Joseph's Hospital in Tampa. At this meeting that I attended, he was presenting Dr. John Shea of Memphis as one of his guest speakers.

During his residency at the Eye and Ear, Dr. Shea became interested in Dr. Jack's attempts to treat deafness by doing a stapedectomy. That surgery, first performed in 1900 at the Eye and Ear, was successful in some cases. However, without the availability of magnification and antibiotics, as I have already stated, several patients died. Dr. Jack discontinued the procedure because of the fatalities that occurred and the storm of criticism by his colleagues. Dr. Shea devoted many months of research and animal dissection before deciding on his approach to a safer surgical procedure. His operation has endured with several different modifications, but the success rate of some 90% has been maintained.

The stapes is the third ossicle of the hearing chain located in the middle ear. The first ossicle to receive the vibrations of sound is the malleus which is attached to the drum. The second ossicle is the incus which carries the vibrations to the third ossicle, the stapes. It is this bone that is affected by the disease called otosclerosis. The footplate of the stapes fits into an opening called the oval window. Otosclerosis causes bone to form around the stapes, preventing it from vibrating and transmitting the sound wave.

John Shea, using a microscope and tiny instruments that he devised, was able to remove the stapes and replace it with a membrane and a plastic tube. The surgery was adopted by ear surgeons in this country and eventually throughout the world.

A Saved Marriage

"Doctor, I'm disappointed in the way my operation turned out."

When Virginia, a thirty-eight-year-old patient made this statement, I was somewhat shocked since there had been no complications following surgery.

I had operated on this lady less than a month before. She had a history of a long-standing hearing loss which had worsened in recent years. One of her close friends was a patient of mine on whom I had performed surgery for deafness. She had an excellent result and referred Virginia and several other friends to me.

Virginia proved to have otosclerosis and was an excellent candidate for stapedectomy. The operation went off successfully. Her postoperative course was uneventful and when I saw her one week later in the office she had improved hearing. I was pleased with the result and told Virginia that further improvement could be expected as the operative swelling diminished.

I examined her again approximately one month after surgery. I found everything in perfect order with excellent hearing in the operated ear and I was puzzled by her complaint of disappointment in her surgery.

"Virginia," I said, "please tell me what's bothering you. Your hearing is excellent and yet you say you're unhappy."

With some tears and and a sad voice, she gave me a full explanation of her problem.

"Doctor, I've been married for nearly twenty years to a wonderful man. As you know I've had this hearing loss ever since I was a teenager. When I went to high school and was fitted with a hearing aid, it was easy to cope with the hearing loss. After graduating from high school I took a job as a secretary and then got married a year later. My work is good and there's no problem with my hearing."

"That all sounds good, Virginia, so what is the difficulty? You can do your office work without thinking about a hearing aid. You can hear sounds like birds singing as soon as you awaken in the morning without having to reach for your hearing aid."

"That's the trouble, Doctor. Before I had the operation I always took the hearing aid out of my ear when I went to bed and I slept soundly. Now I can't sleep in the same room with my husband."

Occasionally patients will have a change in their sleep pattern after undergoing surgery or an illness, but this didn't seem like a reasonable explanation for this problem to develop during the four weeks since surgery.

"I'm not sure if I understand you correctly. Why can't you sleep in the same room with your husband since your surgery?"

"My husband snores and he makes so much noise that he keeps me awake all night. Without a good night's rest I can't stay awake on my job the next day. I've tried going to another room, but that only makes my husband mad. All during our marriage I never realized that he snored because I always removed my hearing aid at bedtime. I couldn't hear those noises he makes, but since the operation they drive me crazy. What can I do?"

Never having had such a problem presented to me before, I was momentarily baffled. I could advise wearing ear plugs to bed so she could block the sounds of snoring, but I decided there had to be a better solution.

Then I recalled when Virginia first came to my office she was accompanied by her husband. He was very interested in the stapedectomy operation I recommended for his wife. He asked a lot of questions as I described the procedure while pointing to a chart on the wall showing the ear and the stapes.

It was quite evident to me that his voice was very nasal and when he blew his nose, which he did quite often, it sounded like a fog horn. This is rather typical of people with a nasal blockage. I naturally made no comment at the time, but now I decided that perhaps there might be a solution for both Virginia and her husband, Jim.

I explained to Virginia why people snore so she would understand the probable cause of his noisy breathing at night. In deep sleep some patients breathe through the mouth, especially if the nasal passages are blocked. The soft palate in the back of the throat flops back and forth like a curtain in the wind. This produces the noise not noticed by the husband but clearly heard by the spouse.

"Virginia, I think that Jim has a nasal blockage that might be correctable. If you can convince him to come into the office someday for an examination, I believe we might be able to do something."

I wasn't sure that I was altogether convincing because Virginia gave me a funny look as if she thought perhaps this doctor has some unusual ideas. She did agree to talk to Jim, but I wasn't very hopeful about the result.

One week later I was pleasantly surprised to see them both in my office. As he sat down in the treatment room chair I had the feeling Jim was making this visit under duress.

"Have you ever had an injury to your nose, Jim?" I began very gently.

"I played a lot of football in high school and got hit in the nose frequently. We didn't have nose guards in those days."

"Do you have any allergies?"

"My nose drips a bit, especially in the summer and fall. And I sneeze occasionally."

An examination of the nose revealed a marked deviation of the septum causing almost a complete blockage of the left side. In addition, there were polyps on both sides which further decreased the airway considerably. These were undoubtedly related to some degree of allergy as confirmed by his history.

At this point Jim admitted using over-the-counter nose drops for many years. He had sought the advice of his family doctor when his breathing became difficult and he got some relief from prescription medication.

Further questioning revealed he was forced to use the nasal spray almost continuously in more recent months. The marked swelling and redness of the nasal mucosa was typical of "nose-drop nose" caused by excessive use of nose drops. In view of the obstruction to his breathing caused by the deviation of the septum and the nasal polyps, I recommended surgery. The septum was straightened out and the polyps excised without difficulty one week later. Two weeks after surgery a pair of happy people presented themselves at my office.

Jim was breathing more comfortably than he had in years and Virginia was enjoying a full night's sleep without being awakened by the loud snoring of her husband.

I felt like a marriage counselor who had just brought two unhappy people joyously together. In this case it was not only the married couple, but also the surgeon who shared in the final successful result.

Hope for the Severely-Deafened Patient

I was impressed by the response of one patient who was presented during a demonstration at St. Vincent's Hospital in Los Angeles. When asked if she felt satisfied by the improvement obtained with her cochlear implant, she replied, "Before my operation I had no privacy."

In the early 1970s a breakthrough occurred that gave some hope to the severely nerve-deafened patient. The pioneering efforts of Dr. William House and others brought about a method of transmitting sound with a cochlear implant.

This implant was designed for patients with severe nerve deafness. In a previous section I described the huge box the patients were forced to use when this operation was first done. Eventually miniaturization allowed the individual to wear all the equipment needed.

There are four components to the cochlear implant: 1. a microphone to pick up the sound waves; 2. a microelectronic system to convert the sound waves into electric signals; 3. a transmission mechanism to relay the electrical signals to implanted components; 4. electrodes going to the auditory nerve.

Several patients who had received these implants were presented by the Otologic Medical group during the week-long seminar in Los Angeles.

The cochlear implant has undergone many modifications since its inception. It is a highly involved technological procedure that required not hours or weeks or months but years of painstaking research. It demands skilled craftsmanship not only by the surgeons, but also the engineers and medical personnel.

When the forty-year-old woman stated that before restoration of her hearing she had no privacy, many in the audience of some 200 ear physicians could not appreciate her reasoning until she explained further:

"When I was alone I had to leave the door open to see who came to my home. Now I keep my door closed and listen for the bell to ring which I can now hear. I then check to see if it's a stranger, the mailman, the delivery person, or a friend who has come to pay a visit. My life has been so deeply enriched I just can't tell you how happy I am."

For those who have never lived in a world of complete silence, this might not be easy to appreciate or understand how profound the loss of sound can be. However, you should allow yourself someday to block off your ears completely so no sound can penetrate. Imagine not hearing the wind blowing through the trees, or the songs of the birds, the ringing of a bell, the sound of a friend's voice, or your child telling you how much she loves you. Only then can you really appreciate why this limited return to the hearing world is such a godsend to the totally deafened person.

We are all acquainted with the miracle of organ transplants such as kidney, heart, liver, lungs, and other body parts. The restoration of hearing to the totally deaf is in its infancy, but amazing progress is being made. Its use in children is just beginning and there is definitely great hope for the future.

BEETLE MANIA

A Flying Bug in the Ear

"Doctor, one of the workers on the golf course has a bug in his ear. Could you see him right away? He says it's driving him crazy."

My office personnel had left for the day. I was off call and looking forward to one of those rare evenings of dinner with the family. When the message came from Mildred Kay, the pro-shop manager, I knew from the urgency in her voice the patient must be in extreme discomfort. However, I also figured there might be a quick and simple solution.

"Call over to the kitchen," I said, "and have one of the help bring you some vegetable oil and pour it into his ear. Then let me know if the man is free of pain."

Judging from past experience I was quite sure the oil would stifle the bug's activity and relieve the worker's discomfort almost immediately. Within a few minutes the phone rang and it was Mrs. Kay again.

"I poured almost a cupful of oil into his ear and he says the pain is getting worse. Should I take him to the emergency room for treatment?"

"No," I said. "It might take quite a while before he's seen. Have someone drive him down to my office and I will get a room set up to take care of him right away."

I called home and told my wife to set my dinner aside.

"It will be another hour before I get home so don't delay the family from eating."

Within a few minutes the patient was in my office. He appeared to be in obvious pain. While positioning him in the treatment chair he described what had happened.

"I was trimming some branches that were loaded with Japanese beetles when all of a sudden I felt one of them go into my ear. I tried to dig it out with my finger but then it started to bite me. The more I tried to remove the bug the worse the pain became."

With the headlight adjusted and a small forceps in my hand, the ear canal was exposed. I inserted the speculum and was now ready to remove the bug. What a surprise! I saw nothing but a huge mass of wax that filled the outer ear canal.

"Herb, you don't have a beetle in your ear," I said. "Your ear is loaded with wax. I don't know how that could've given you all that pain. Let me get the wax out and your troubles will be over."

A quick squirt of water from the ear syringe and a few moments later a large glob of wax fell into the basin.

Almost triumphantly I announced, "There's your problem, Herb. You must have had that blockage for a long time."

"But Doctor," Herb protested, "my ear has never felt blocked and the pain is still there and now seems worse than ever."

I looked into the ear and couldn't see the drum. The whole canal except for the outer edge was markedly edematous and inflamed. The swelling had been covered up by the wax I had just removed.

"Herb, your ear canal is so completely blocked off I can't see the drum. Let's go into the microscope room. Perhaps I can force a small ear tube through that swollen area and see what is happening."

Over the years the operating microscope proved to be one of my best instruments. With some difficulty I was finally able to get my smallest cone-shaped ear speculum through the swollen canal.

Staring back at me through the microscope were the menacing eyes of a bug. Beyond those eyes was the green and brown spotted body of what I was now able to identify as a Japanese beetle. It was thrashing about and beating up against the drum which was edematous and beefy red.

"Herb, it will only take a few minutes more. I have the bug cornered. First I'll put him to sleep and that will stop his biting."

A squirt of ethyl chloride anesthesia stopped the bug's activity and gave my patient immediate relief of his pain. There was no possible way to remove the entire beetle in one piece through the narrow ear speculum. I first cut the legs with the dissecting scissors and removed them. I did the same thing with the wings. After the head was removed it was necessary to cut up the huge body and remove it piece by piece. Although all this bug dissection took almost ten minutes Herb had no further pain. Once the bug had been knocked out by the anesthetic spray there was no further agonizing pain from the drum being bitten.

I now reviewed the sequence of events with Herb.

"When that insect hit your ear," I said, "you did the obvious thing. You put your finger in your ear and tried to get it out. Instead of getting it out you pushed the beetle deeper into the ear between the wax and the canal. The beetle kept biting the canal wall as it was being pushed inward towards the drum. Once it got into the space between the drum and the wax you really started to feel the pain. That's when the beetle went to work on the drum while trying to get out of captivity."

Finally I gave Herb on piece of advice:

"Since you frequently work in areas infested with Japanese beetles, it would be a good idea if you wore some kind of ear protection. That should prevent any bug from getting into your ear."

The next day Herb phoned to say he was feeling fine. Since the tissue diagnosis was obvious, I didn't bother having the pathology department identify the bug as a Japanese beetle. Instead I put the segments of the insect into a small container and mailed it to the patient. I included a note stating the unusual sequence of events that occurred helped to make history of sorts and would also make an unbelievable story to tell his friends.

Japanese beetles came from Japan originally, as you would expect. They devour leaves, fruits, and grasses and are damaging to crops. They are prevalent during the warm seasons especially in the northeast. They have become a real nuisance on the golf courses to which they seem to be attracted.

If one flies into your ear, a frequent occurrence, the bite is painful and is doubly so when it attacks the drum. Ordinarily the best treatment is vegetable oil, but if that's not immediately available then use water. However, unlike some insects the beetle can float around in a watery medium and continue to cause pain and discomfort.

Under any circumstances don't attempt to dig it out or ask a friend to do so. That could be disastrous.

A Golfer and a Japanese Beetle

A fellow golfer and next-door neighbor leaned over the fence and said, "I heard you removed a beetle from a guy's ear who works on the the golf course."

"That's right, Bill, but it wasn't easy."

"I was going to call you this afternoon, Doctor, but everything worked out OK."

My curiosity was aroused. "What happened?"

"We were playing the 12th hole when my partner, Jim Smith, started to jump up and down. He put a finger in his ear and yelled that one of those damn Japanese beetles was flying around as he was putting. He tried to brush it away, but it went into his ear. It started to bite him and he asked me to try to get it out."

"What did you do then, Bill?" I asked.

"I looked in his ear and told him I couldn't see a damn thing. Then Jim asked me to put a golf tee into his ear and dig out the bug."

"Don't tell me you did that, Bill," I said, shaking my head in disbelief.

"Well actually, I had a wooden tee in my hand and was going to put that in his ear when he said the bug had flown out."

"Putting a golf tee into his ear would've been the worst thing you could have done, Bill, since you can't see inside the canal and could have ruptured the ear drum. If you meet with this problem again the quickest thing to do is try some water out of the brook, even a soda might be used. That may cut down the biting for a while."

"What then?" Bill asked.

"If it's still bothering the golfer you'd better head for the emergency room to have it removed. You might want to stop at the club house and try some vegetable oil in the ear if the bug is still biting."

A Missionary's Earwax Makes Medical History

"Father Murphy," I said, "you have enough wax in your ears to make a candle."

My patient had just returned from China where he had started his missionary life many years before. For several months he had noted increasing difficulty in hearing which was undoubtedly related to the wax I now observed. While gathering my instruments to remove the cerumen, Father Murphy began an interesting story of his life in the Orient.

"From the early days of my priesthood one of my primary objectives was to become a missionary. After being ordained I volunteered for duty first in the Philippines, then for assignment to China. It was a short time later that the communists gained control and all the clergy, both foreign and Chinese, were arrested and put on trial and incarcerated."

Father Murphy paused and then started to relate the problems that developed.

"Several years later I was released from prison and placed under house arrest. This allowed me a certain amount of liberty, but conduction of religious services was strictly forbidden."

This kindly, soft-spoken, sixty-year-old priest exhibited no bitterness as he recounted some of his experiences.

"My missionary order, the Maryknolls, was given permission to send me a small amount of money for my maintenance. The room where I lived was sufficient for my bed and my stove for cooking."

While he spoke Father Murphy interjected his words with an occasional laugh and said nothing of the mental torment he undoubtedly suffered. His inability to give spiritual guidance or saying mass for his Christian followers was admittedly disturbing to this dedicated man. The majority of ordained Jews, Protestants, and Catholics all seem to tolerate religious persecutions better than most of us endure our daily hardships.

After mentioning the amount of wax I saw in his ears, Father Murphy remarked, "I'll never forget the problems which we encountered when wax had to be purchased for making candles. I bought the wax in the large market place where most household products were sold."

I stopped my preparations for cleaning out his ear and asked, "How did you ever learn to make the candles?"

"That was no problem, but buying the wax occasionally caused some difficulties. This candle-making material was rolled into a round ball usually weighing up to several pounds or more. Naturally the weight of the wax determined the charge."

Father Murphy hesitated a moment, smiling as his thoughts came flooding back.

"You had to be careful," he said, "since some of the merchants were unscrupulous and wouldn't hesitate to stuff a stone into the center of the wax increasing the weight and of course your cost. Sometimes you wouldn't know you had been cheated by the dealer until you returned to your quarters and started to make the candles. When you cut into the ball of wax you discovered the stone and realized then you had been swindled without any recourse. After one such experience I always insisted on cutting through the ball of wax. I wanted to make sure I wasn't going to be cheated again. The proprietor would usually become excited and angry because of my demand, especially since I was one of those foreign devils as he called me."

While irrigating the left ear I stood there fascinated by this interesting story as related by this most congenial missionary. A large clump of wax fell into the basin with complete relief of the blockage.

"That feels a lot better," Father Murphy said, "but the right ear has given me trouble for a longer period of time."

"Don't worry, Father," I said. "We'll fix the right ear in the same way."

I spoke too soon. The irrigating syringe was filled with water not once but three times and still the wax didn't move.

"The wax in the right ear won't budge," I said. "I'll have to use the hook method to get it out since this wax is really solid."

By maneuvering my instrument around the mass I was able to move it forward finally. I then inspected the ball of material after I placed it in the specimen basin. All I could say was "I'll be damned."

Beneath the thin veneer of the wax ball I had removed was a solid interior of stony material. I immediately recalled attending an ENT meeting in Atlantic City several months earlier. At that time, Dr. Arthur Proetz, a distinguished otolaryngologist from St. Louis reported a case of an otolith, only the second such recorded in fifty years of the prestigious Triological Society.

"Father Murphy, your story of checking the purchase of wax for an implanted stone was unusual, to say the least. This stone formation in your ear is even more unusual because it's such a rare event. You have made medical history."

My clinical diagnosis of otolith, stone formation in the ear, was confirmed by the pathology department at the hospital. Searching the medical literature failed to uncover any other cases of otoliths except for the report of Dr. Proetz.

Father Murphy's wax purchase experience in China, followed by the true life incident of this rare phenomenon in his ear, made me realize that in medicine, truth is certainly stranger than fiction.

14
Swallowing Problems in Children

Baby Chokes on Carrot

This headline in the Hartford newspaper caught my eye as I was scanning the headlines. The young mother, whose name I recognized immediately, had recently been a patient of mine. According to the paper's account the mother had just returned from a shopping trip. She placed her two-year-old daughter in the playpen and at that same moment the phone rang.

The mother hastily gave the child one of the carrots which she had purchased for the evening meal and then went into the next room to answer the call.

She returned to the kitchen in a few minutes and found the infant blue and motionless. The child had chewed off a piece of the carrot which she apparently attempted to swallow. The vegetable became lodged in her throat blocking her breathing passage causing asphyxia and death. The frantic mother called the emergency number of the police who responded immediately, but the youngster couldn't be revived.

One of the more common emergencies encountered by the ENT specialist occurs when food is caught in the throat.

Children and often adults attempt to swallow food which isn't thoroughly chewed or something is placed in the mouth, like a toy, that doesn't belong there. Occasionally the adult has a loose-fitting denture which becomes dislodged and ends up as an emergency operative procedure.

Small children, especially two years or under, shouldn't be given nuts, popcorn, or hard to chew raw vegetables such as carrots. At this age their teeth have not always been developed to grind these materials so they can safely enter into the food passage. This kind of hard material can quickly cause obstruction by becoming embedded in the upper food passage (the pharynx) where it presses against the airway. It's a tragic sequence of events that far too often ends in the death of the youngster.

Chasing the Glass Aggie

"What do you think about this, Dr. Curran?"

The pediatric resident put up an admission chest film on the x-ray screen which showed a globular object located in the upper part of the esophagus.

"What is it and how did it get there?" I said.

"This is a three-year-old Puerto Rican boy," the resident said, "who was in good health until three days ago. At dinner time he was unable to take anything by mouth except fluids. When solid foods were taken they were immediately vomited."

"What happened then?" I asked.

"Apparently no amount of coaxing by the mother could encourage little Francisco to swallow anything except milk and soda. Today she decided to bring him to the hospital."

With a high percentage of emergency patients who speak only Spanish, the hospital always has an attendant who acts as an interpreter. This Spanish-speaking individual was asked to get a more complete story from the mother who was in the waiting room.

The interpreter reported back after a few minutes

"Francisco had been playing a game of aggies with his two brothers just before mealtime. The two older boys put the glass balls in their mouths while playing and Francisco apparently did the same thing. He showed no signs of choking at any time, but when he put food in his mouth it was vomited almost immediately. He did drink soda without any difficulty, but no amount of scolding could get him to take food after the first few efforts."

"Usually such a smooth rounded object will make its way into the stomach and eventually be passed without incident," I said to the resident. "But apparently this foreign body is too large to pass through this child's esophagus. It's location just behind the windpipe may eventually cause obstruction to his breathing, therefore, the glass aggie should be removed immediately by endoscopy. First, I want you to contact the mother and have her bring in all the children's aggies. We need to find one that is the the exact size of the glass ball we see in the x-ray."

That afternoon we found the exact duplicate from the children's collection. Dr. Sennett in the x-ray department found the size of the ball in the film to be one-half inch in diameter.

After checking the supply cabinet of instruments in the operating room I knew our troubles were not yet over. The duplicate aggie that I had couldn't be encircled by any of the forceps among our OR supplies.

It looked as though the removal could only be accomplished by having one of the surgeons open up the chest.

Retracing my steps toward the pediatric floor I met Danny Donahue, a key employee at the hospital. He was recognized as a master carpenter and jack of all trades.

He stopped and asked, "What's wrong, Doc? You look worried."

"I am worried, Danny," I said, "and this is the reason."

Danny knew all about our instruments in the operating room where he spent considerable time building shelves and repairing surgical chairs among many other duties. He readily understood my problem when I talked to him about taking out foreign bodies using the esophagoscope and forceps.

I pulled out the glass aggie and described the problem facing me.

"My main concern," I said, "is not having an instrument to reach down through my scope to grasp a marble of this size that's blocking off the youngster's swallowing."

There was no hesitancy on Danny's part as he responded immediately.

"Let's go over to the engineering department," he said. "I think we may have something you can use."

Danny's workshop was filled with all kinds of gadgets. He brought me over to one corner where there was a large chest with many drawers.

"OK, Doc, here you are," he said proudly. "There must be something in there you can use on that kid."

The assortment of tools temporarily baffled me as Danny explained, "These tools are used to reach down and retrieve objects that have fallen into water tanks."

Some of the metal devices were five feet long and three to four inches wide, but there were other claws, as they were called, that were six to twelve inches long and narrow enough to fit through an operating esophagoscope. With Danny's help we found a few of these implements that would not only grasp the glass aggie in my hand but might also fit through the esophagoscope.

After thanking Danny I rushed up to the doctors' lounge of the operating room where I scrubbed the water-tank claws until they looked almost presentable. Entering the cabinet room where the esophagoscopes were stored, I found the child-size tube that would allow the insertion of my newly-acquired instrument.

At that moment Nora Walsh, the OR supervisor, came by and in a somewhat demanding manner asked, "What are you doing here with those cruddy-looking instruments in your hands?"

"Nora, I have a three-year-old patient," I said, "who swallowed an aggie which is stuck in his esophagus. None of our instruments can grab that glass marble, but this tool can do the trick."

While saying this I held up the claw.

"This new tool will not only hold the aggie, but also will fit through the pediatric esophagoscope we'll use."

Nora came right back at me.

"How do you know that this harebrained idea of yours will work?"

"Nora, there's no other way we can remove this glass aggie unless you want to have this child undergo major surgery."

That was the convincer and she finally agreed to book the endoscopy for the following morning.

Little Francisco was receiving intravenous fluids when I visited him later and he was showing no ill effects from the aggie lodged in his esophagus.

X-rays were again taken since imbedded objects occasionally start to move down into the stomach after being delayed for several days. The glass marble was in the same exact position. Nothing could be gained by delaying the endoscopy.

The next day our little patient was placed under anesthesia and the esophagoscope inserted to the approximate level where the aggie was located which was previously determined to be ten centimeters from the upper teeth. The newly acquired tool, now sterilized and called an operating forceps, was inserted through the scope with a firm expectation that the object of my search would be seen and successful surgery could be accomplished.

However, much to my surprise I didn't see the aggie.

"Perhaps the anesthesia has relaxed the muscles enough," I said to the anesthetist, "to allow the aggie to move into the stomach and then be passed naturally. Let's get another x-ray here in the operating room and see what's happened."

In a short time the x-rays were taken and I was surprised again. The glass marble had not changed its position one millimeter. The esophagoscope was again introduced and at the measured level from the upper jaw I rubbed the forceps up against the pink mucosa.

At that point I exclaimed, "I think I've found it."

Within seconds after pushing the delicate tissues aside, I identified the glass aggie clearly. I opened the mouth of the forceps and easily encircled it and then withdrew it from the boy's esophagus carefully in one quick motion.

The glass aggie proved to be the exact color as the esophageal tissues and not green or yellow or orange as the marbles that the mother had brought in for my inspection. My childhood remembrance of aggies had failed to recall all the colors.

Francisco was discharged the following day after I watched him happily consume his first meal in four days.

The OR supervisor, Miss Walsh, decided that more appropriate instruments should be obtained from the surgical supply house so we wouldn't have to depend on any Rube Goldberg facsimiles. The new forceps were ordered and certainly looked more attractive, but weren't necessarily anymore effective than those rescued from the confines of the engineer's treasure trove.

The claw that saved the day was returned to its proper environment and I congratulated Danny Donahue for helping to make the operation a success.

"You deserve a reward for your help, Danny," I said, patting him on the back. "And I'm going to split the fee with you which consists of the deep gratitude of the patient and his mother."

Some years later a fee schedule was set up through the welfare service to reimburse the doctor for his care of the indigent. It never seemed to give quite the same joy that was often experienced when there was no monetary return but pure gratitude instead.

A Broken Spring — A Failed Surgery

While making rounds in the morning the pediatric resident, Dr. Allen, mentioned an interesting case of a five-year-old youngster whose mother said he had been experiencing a severe cough for several days.

"Shortly after admission to our pediatric service," the resident continued, "we asked Dr. Bowen, the chest consultant, to see the patient. When he reviewed the x-rays, which showed a screw in the right lung, he said that it could be removed by bronchoscopy. That operation was done yesterday, but he was unable to remove the foreign body."

Dr. Bowen was a chest physician who had privileges for diagnostic bronchoscopy which limited his treatment to diseases of the lungs. With no surgical training or experience he didn't have privileges for removal of foreign bodies.

"What does Dr. Bowen suggest?" I asked Dr. Allen.

"He wants the general surgeon, Dr. Ellis, to see the patient for lung surgery."

This case now became of greater interest to me since any patient with a foreign body in the lung is the responsibility of the nose and throat endoscopic service.

"Let's go down to the radiology department," I said to Dr. Allen. "I'd like to review those films."

Dr. Sennett, the radiologist, put the films up on the view box.

"As you can see," he said, "the screw is located in the entrance of the bronchus leading to the upper lobe of the right lung."

"It's not possible," I said, "to turn the bronchoscope into the upper lobe bronchus which, as you know, is at a right angle from the main tract of the lung. How can I see and grasp the screw even with an angulated forceps?"

Dr. Sennett offered a suggestion.

"We might have a solution for that with a new piece of equipment. It's a television camera attachment allowing the surgeon to use his instrument while watching the TV screen. You don't need to look through the bronchoscope to see where you're going. Everything is done while watching the screen."

This was really interesting and I immediately said, "Tell me more."

We went into the room that was set up with the TV camera. The equipment was turned on and a mannequin was used to demonstrate how the operation could be done.

I called Dr. Ellis and reminded him that proper protocol hadn't been observed when the case was turned over to him.

"Furthermore," I added, "Bronchoscopy may avoid the necessity of opening up the chest of this five-year-old child. If it doesn't work then I'll call you to do the chest surgery."

During my ENT residency training I gained considerable experience in endoscopic procedures. I supplemented that training with a one-month course given by Chevalier Jackson at his world-renowned clinic in Philadelphia. This advanced instruction which I took before I formally started my private practice gave me an opportunity to learn the latest techniques developed during the war.

The television screen connected to the bronchoscope would give me visual access to the screw in the lung. However, I needed an instrument to grasp the foreign body. After obtaining a matching screw from engineering, I checked our instrument cabinet. A right-angle forceps was found that would clamp onto the screw I had in my hand. Conceivably this delicate instrument could reach in and remove the screw since the location of the upper lobe bronchus wouldn't allow contact with a straight forceps.

The day before the surgery the whole procedure was practiced on the mannequin using the TV with the angle forceps and the duplicate screw. After speaking with Dr. Scully, the anesthesiologist, he became just as excited as I was about this innovative procedure.

The next day our patient, Manuel, was wheeled down to the x-ray department and readied for the surgery. He proved to be a cooperative patient and after a few minutes Dr. Scully announced: "The patient is ready and you can start the operation."

As I inserted the bronchoscope the whole procedure was easily visualized on the television screen by the radiologist, the anesthesiologist, the nurse assistant, and me. I worked the bronchoscope toward the upper lobe of the right lung and guided the forceps towards the screw. All of this was accomplished while watching the television screen.

The bronchoscope couldn't enter into the angulated right bronchus where the metallic foreign body was located. However, it was easy to follow the direction of the small right-angle forceps as I turned it and made immediate contact with the screw.

I placed the forceps on the screw and was just about to withdraw it from the lung when Dr. Scully suddenly cried out, "Stop everything! The child isn't breathing."

Quickly loosening my hold on the foreign body, I pulled out the bronchoscope and the forceps. The child had become cyanotic, but after a few minutes of oxygen the anesthesia was restarted and Dr. Scully gave me the reassuring words: "He's OK now and you can resume the operation."

I reinserted the bronchoscope and once again using the TV screen as a visual guide, I came into contact with the elusive screw. However, all attempts to grasp it failed to make it budge.

As everyone looked on with great expectation, I finally had to say, "There's something wrong and I can't figure out what it is. My forceps won't grab onto the screw even though as you can see contact is being made. I may have to quit."

After several more unsuccessful efforts, I withdrew the forceps to check the cause of the difficulty. It was then I discovered the forcep's spring was broken which prevented its teeth from closing on the screw.

After thoroughly inspecting the forceps I realized it couldn't be fixed. Resigned to this unfortunate circumstance, I turned to Dr. Scully and asked him to stop the anesthesia.

I called Dr. Ellis later. He agreed to perform the chest surgery the following day. The screw was removed along with the upper lobe of the right lung. Young Manuel was discharged from the hospital two weeks later. We all realized that he would encounter some disability with the partial loss of his right lung.

The early days of endoscopic surgery were full of such frustrations as having an inadequate supply of proper instruments. This was especially true of some of the unusual cases that were seen on occasions.

During this pioneering period many lives were saved and major operative procedures were often avoided by performing endoscopy. However, the occasional embarrassment of failure was an added impetus to have backup instruments in our cabinet of endoscopic equipment.

The failure to achieve success in removing the screw reminded me of the well-known aphorism: "For want of a nail the shoe was lost."

A Pea Bean in the Lung

Billy was an active six-year-old boy who had found great pleasure with a new toy he had acquired. It was called a pea-bean shooter.

"Look Mom, watch this."

After demonstrating his prowess inside the house it became evident Billy was messing up the walls, the floor, and the furniture. His mother decided his indoor activity should be carried on outside.

It was some weeks later that Billy went out with his shooter, but within minutes came back dashing into the house. He was coughing and gagging to such a point he was unable to talk.

He finally quieted down enough to give an explanation to his worried mother.

"I put some peas in my mouth," he said, "and started to blow them across the street at the lamp post. Some of them got caught in my throat and made me cough."

His mother was not too concerned at first, but Billy continued to cough rather violently. She decided to call the pediatrician who advised her that her son should be further checked at the emergency room. The pediatrician called me at home as I was enjoying a relaxing Saturday afternoon. He explained what had happened.

Before Billy arrived at the hospital I called the emergency room and alerted the supervisor.

"Ask the x-ray department to take a film of the chest. Don't allow the child to have anything by mouth. It may be necessary to bronchoscope him."

The pediatrician and I arrived at the hospital shortly after Billy came to the emergency room. Our patient appeared comfortable and wasn't coughing.

The chest x-rays showed no signs of a foreign body. However, the pea bean isn't radio-opaque and won't always show up as a shadow on the film. The pediatrician placed a stethoscope on Billy's chest and then turned to me.

"Billy has some wheezing on the right side. What do you think we should do, Tim?"

"Even though the films are negative, I'd advise a bronchoscopy. It's possible the pea bean is stuck down there, probably in the right lung where you hear the wheezing. This could cause a problem sometime in the future, maybe weeks or months from now."

Billy was brought to the operating room where he was placed under anesthesia. Having had no food for several hours, it wasn't necessary to delay the operation.

Following insertion of the bronchoscope I immediately saw a pea in the right bronchus and removed it without difficulty. Most foreign bodies end up in the right side of the lung when they are sucked in from the throat. The right bronchus is on a direct line from the trachea above. I also examined the left bronchus, but as I anticipated this area was clear.

The aspiration of material from the mouth into the lungs isn't uncommon in children. This also occurs occasionally in adults. Talking and especially laughing while eating may produce the inhalation effect. In most cases the coughing that develops will expel the foreign body. But if there is any question, then bronchoscopy should be performed.

If a foreign body remains in the lung it usually sets up a reaction in the tissues. This may develop into an infection resulting in pneumonia or a collapsed lung several months or more after the incident.

Billy was discharged the following morning and the parents assured me the pea shooter would no longer be included in his assortment of toys.

The Death of Juanita

I reviewed the film in the x-ray department and then turned to the pediatric interne who was at my elbow.

"How did the pin get in there?" I said.

The x-ray showed the outline of an open safety pin in the upper esophagus.

"We don't know how or when it found its way into the esophagus, Dr. Curran," the interne said. "Juanita is a thirteen-month-old child who was born at the local home for unwed mothers. The young mother has another small baby at home and is unable to take care of this child. She's been under the care of the nuns from birth since like so many other black children, adoption rarely takes place."

"How long has the pin been caught up in there? Do you know?"

"We don't know the exact time, but a week ago Juanita became listless and failed to take her nourishment except for limited amounts of fluids. A few days later she was showing tarry-colored stools which continued for several more days when the pediatric consultant was asked to examine the baby. He advised laboratory examinations including blood tests that showed a markedly low count. Hospitalization was advised and the admission chest x-ray showed the open safety pin in the esophagus."

The interne, Dr. Kelly, continued to look at the film and then turned to me.

"How can the pin be removed, Dr. Curran?"

"The pin has to be removed by esophagoscopy, but it'll be difficult since the point is facing upward and is obviously imbedded in the tissues. If the keeper of the pin is grasped with the forceps any forceful movement upward will only push the pin deeper into the tissues. This will cause a lot of bleeding as the pin tears into the tissues. The chances are the pin can't be released in that position."

"How can it be taken out then?"

I asked one of the technicians to get me a safety pin. With the safety pin in my hand I demonstrated how the procedure would be done.

"When the pin is seen through the scope, I'll grasp it with the forceps by the coiled end and push it into the stomach. In the stomach it can be turned around so the point will be facing downward. Once that is done the scope can be withdrawn dragging the forceps and the attached pin behind it."

"But," I cautioned, "nothing can be attempted until Juanita's blood count is improved with a transfusion of whole blood."

I checked the operating room's instrument cabinet. All the proper equipment was available for the surgery. It took several days of transfusions before the pediatrician agreed Juanita's condition could withstand the anesthesia and surgery.

Despite all the precautions I had a great deal of concern as to the likelihood of further bleeding during the procedure. Although it appeared there was no active bleeding at this time, any blood clot in the esophagus could give way and further hemorrhage might occur. Several large syringes of blood were ordered for instant transfusion, if needed.

After Juanita had been placed under anesthesia, I carefully introduced the scope into the esophagus down to the level where I saw the safety pin. I then inserted the forceps and attached it to the coiled end.

"Be ready with that blood if we need it. I'm going to move the pin towards the stomach now and we may run into some bleeding. So far everything looks good."

Once in the stomach cavity the pin easily turned and the point was now facing downwards.

"I am going to pull up the scope now and the forceps with the attached pin should follow right behind it. So far I can't see any bleeding."

The scope, forceps, and pin were brought out of the mouth and the pin was dropped into the specimen basin. I had a great feeling of triumph with the success of my effort when suddenly a gush of blood came spewing from the child's mouth.

"Quick, give me that narrow gauze packing we have ready. I've got to stop this bleeding immediately. There's no way I can see the exact point of hemorrhage otherwise."

As I pushed the gauze packing into the esophagus the anesthesiologist called for the syringes of blood to be started. In about fifteen long minutes the pulse and the blood pressure began to normalize and I slowly removed the packing. For another thirty minutes we all waited anxiously, hoping there wouldn't be any further bleeding. At the end of that time it was agreed Juanita could be returned to her room on the pediatric floor.

Several hours later she developed a croupy cough and the pediatrician had her placed in the croup room. For three days her breathing continued to be somewhat labored. Gradually her condition improved and it now appeared as if our little patient was going to make a complete recovery.

While I walked toward the croup room on the fifth postoperative day, the nurse greeted me with a big smile and good news.

"The pediatrician just examined Juanita," she said, "and her croup has cleared and she can be transferred back to the general pediatric ward."

I followed the nurse into the room, sharing her happiness.

"She had me worried for awhile," I said, "but it looks as though she has now turned the corner."

When we reached Juanita's crib, the nurse turned the infant toward us and we saw that her lips were blue.

The nurse screamed, "She's not breathing! I think she's dead."

I quickly placed a stethoscope on the little child's chest. I couldn't hear any heart beat or any breath sounds. While I began resuscitation I told the nurse to call the inhalation team, but I had the sinking feeling all our efforts were ending in disaster. Despite the help of the anesthesiologists and other supporting groups who had come instantly, Juanita couldn't be resuscitated.

The autopsy showed a clot deep within the wall of the esophagus near the original point of the pin penetration. It was determined that this clot was pressing against the adjacent vagus nerve which controls the heart beat. The blood clot probably had first caused some interference with the adjacent recurrent nerve controlling the vocal cords. Undoubtedly this nerve pressure had produced the croupy breathing noted shortly after surgery.

Based on the pathologist's report, Juanita's death was attributed to cardiac failure. After reviewing the events following the child's admission to the hospital many questions came to my mind as to why all these events took place.

What could have been done to prevent this tragedy before the pin found its way into the esophagus? What different approach, if any, could have been attempted to safely remove the pin and preserve the life of this little child?

There was never any reasonable explanation as to how an infant of Juanita's age could find an open safety pin and place it in her mouth and swallow it. That mystery was never solved.

In preparing our little patient for surgery every precaution was taken to insure a successful result. This included the selection of proper instruments, repeat x-rays, blood control, and pediatric consultation. Everything went along as planned with all the protective mechanisms being initiated as soon as the complications of bleeding occurred. Even the unexpected development of croup appeared to be under control when death suddenly intervened.

In reviewing the tragic course of events I developed my own scenario of what may have happened. Juanita was a lovable, smiling child and this was especially evident during her recovery from surgery. She was always reaching out her little arms to those who came into the croup room.

The croup area usually had three or four patients who were visited daily by members of their families. They gave these children all the affection and warmth that Juanita certainly yearned for, but usually in vain. Only the nurses and the other medical personnel were available to respond to her outstretched arms. However, they were limited in their ability and desire to give Juanita all the needed attention because of the care being given to other patients.

There were no visitors and no family who came to cuddle Juanita and make her feel wanted and loved. Perhaps the diagnosis of cardiac failure rendered by the pathologist was anatomically correct, but another diagnosis could also be developed: "Death due to a broken heart which no one could repair except a loving parent or family."

Juanita had none of this support during her short time on earth. Her outlook for the future might have been cloudy, but who could predict what might have happened if our attempts to save her life had been successful?

15
SWALLOWING PROBLEMS IN ADULTS

A Family Experience with Choking

"Throw her over the table, Tim, or she'll choke to death."

My wife and my sister and her husband had joined our two California cousins for a farewell dinner in San Francisco before departing eastward the next day.

Suddenly Ann, our sixty-four-year-old cousin, started to gag and cough in a croup-like fashion as she stood up gasping for air. Her sister Kathleen cried out that this had happened before and the tabletop was the only place to bring relief.

The dishes with the partially-finished meal would have to be swept to the floor for immediate clearance of the table if I planned to follow Kathleen's suggestion. However, I wasn't convinced Kathleen's suggested treatment was the best solution for the emergency.

I moved quickly to Ann's side. My first thought was where could I procure a knife sharp enough to make an incision in her neck and trachea and relieve the obstruction in her airway?

The apprehension of the family was by now shared by the other diners at the surrounding tables as many stood up and riveted their attention first on Ann and then on me as I stood by her side.

I gently rubbed her back and reassured her that her discomfort was going to be relieved very shortly. Kathleen in the meantime continued to cry out "Throw her over the table, Tim, throw her over the table."

After gesturing to the others that they should sit down, I put a finger to my lips indicating they must remain silent. The past history of choking revealed by Kathleen convinced me this was a spasm that would subside in a few minutes. The victim's apprehension is always increased by the vocal anxiety of the other dinner companions.

The back rub was only to let her know I was close by, thereby helping to lessen her tension. This reassurance would decrease the spasm that was holding the lump of food against her airway. In a few moments Ann's breathing returned to normal and complete calm returned to our table as we silently finished our meal. Ann restricted her intake to fluids.

The Heimlich maneuver which was described some fifteen years later in 1974 is basically the same approach that was recommended by Kathleen when she repeatedly told me to throw her over the table.

When the choking person lies face down over the table, there is pressure on the lower part of the chest and stomach which helps to expel the impacted food from the throat. Heimlich's approach was more effective, being backed by scientific research and animal experiments. Kathleen Kelly's observation should have prompted me to follow up on her suggestion by some investigation of my own.

I did advise Ann to have a checkup by a gastroenterologist who was later consulted. He found a small diverticulum (a pouching out) of her esophagus where food would collect and precipitate symptoms such as she experienced. He told her surgery was unnecessary, but the intake of very small portions of food would minimize a recurrence of her problem.

Alcohol wasn't associated with Ann's intake difficulties since she was a lifetime teetotaler. As commonly known, over-indulgence in alcoholic beverages frequently precedes the choking spell. The resultant impaction of the unchewed piece of beef produces the blockage of the airway and subsequent death of the victim.

Cafe Coronary Syndrome

"Why have so many heart attacks occurred at this one dining place, especially involving victims in their 30s and 40s? This isn't an age when heart attacks are very likely to occur."

A very inquisitive coroner raised this interesting question shortly after his appointment to this investigative position in the city of Miami.

The relationship of over-imbibing, choking, and death, usually while eating steak was brought to the attention of the medical community in the late 1950s. A number of diners had died following "heart attacks" at a well-known restaurant in Miami, Florida.

Careful investigation by the coroner's office revealed that the involved eating place had established a reputation for serving not only the best and tastiest steaks in town, but also dispensing the biggest and driest martinis. This was an attraction that wasn't easily challenged by competitors, but the fatal combination brought a trail of death as determined by the coroner.

The new coroner performed autopsies on a number of victims whose death had previously been attributed to heart attacks. He reported his findings and conclusions as follows:

"The cause of death in many exhumed bodies wasn't due to a heart attack but an obstructing piece of meat which produced asphyxia."

The new coroner had the intuition and the persistence of an investigative detective as he sought out the details of the events leading to the misdiagnosed deaths. He reviewed the events.

"The fatal incidents occurred usually during a heavy-drinking party. When the victim became unconscious the other members of the party weren't fully aware of what had happened. An emergency call was routinely sent out for a physician who examined and pronounced the death of the patient. His information of the circumstances leading to the death was given to him by the proprietor of the restaurant. The physician, under the circumstances, found no reason to suspect death due to choking on food since none of the members in the party were aware of the victim gagging."

As a follow-up on this somewhat challenging inquiry, the coroner established a protocol for deaths under his jurisdiction. It required that all individuals whose deaths were diagnosed as heart attacks during the time of eating should be subjected to autopsy. This strong legal advice was initially aimed at the restaurant where the unusual numbers of so-called heart attacks had occurred, but eventually included all public facilities in the city.

After publication of the Miami coroner's report, other physicians became alerted to the possibility of a death occurring under similar circumstances. Within a few months the incidence of fatalities or near-death from obstructive food intake, especially meat, was reported from all parts of the country. Deaths undoubtedly will continue to occur from such a cause despite the warnings, but the legal requirement of autopsy examination will more correctly identify why the victim expired.

In most communities of our country the laws for verification of the cause of sudden or unexplained death now require an autopsy to be performed. The inclusion of private gatherings, including homes, has helped to publicize the necessity of alerting everyone that alcoholic intake combined with the intake of food such as beef could precipitate a fatality. It also created an interest in developing a method of saving lives with a technique that could be used by anybody, even non-physicians. This is, as I mentioned previously, the Heimlich maneuver.

The coroner published his article as "The Cafe Coronary Syndrome." In view of the developments that occurred before and after the author took office, the title of the paper he wrote was most apt and descriptive.

The Heimlich Hug

In 1975, a Cincinnati surgeon reported his results in removing obstructing pieces of meat from the throats of people who were choking. It became known as the "Heimlich Hug." Dr. Heimlich had described this procedure after many months of animal research and the successful treatment of patients.

It was accomplished by forcing air from the lungs which in turn pushed the obstruction out of the airway. The Heimlich Hug is done by grasping the patient below the chest and squeezing the upper abdominal wall. This will produce the air necessary to dislodge the impacted piece of meat. There's no doubt that this manipulation has saved lives although the indications for doing the procedure is often questionable.

An acquaintance of mine with no training in the technique boasted that he has successfully performed the maneuver; a celebrated news commentator was credited with saving the life of a dinner companion; these anecdotal stories lend a good deal of support to those who claim similar success in doing the so-called hug on strangers and friends.

A gastroenterologist was called one evening to attend a patient who had been admitted to the hospital. The young man apparently had a choking spell while eating meat in a local restaurant. The obstructing piece of beef was causing discomfort, but wasn't life-threatening and was easily removed by the doctor. The patient was discharged from the hospital several hours later.

The next morning the local newspaper ran a headline report about the life-saving Heimlich procedure performed by a truck driver who was in the restaurant on that particular evening. There wasn't any mention of the fact the same patient had been admitted to the hospital where a doctor actually relieved the victim of his discomfort.

Many individuals have experienced a gagging sensation when food becomes temporarily caught in their throats. Although such an event can produce asphyxia and loss of life, the discomfort is best relieved by avoiding panic and admitting the patient to the hospital for proper care. If the patient can't talk and is unable to breathe, the Heimlich Hug may be attempted as described above. Before this is done there should be mouth to mouth breathing along with pressure on the chest.

The Heimlich maneuver isn't a simple procedure. The forceful pressure by strong but untrained individuals has caused the fracture of ribs with puncture of the lungs when it has been attempted in some choking victims. A gagging, uncomfortable person isn't necessarily someone who is at death's door.

There are a few things that shouldn't be done. First and foremost, bystanders should resist the temptation "to do something."

Turning the patients upside down, slapping them on the back, or putting a finger down the throat to remove the blockage shouldn't be done. That heroic but misguided gesture may cause the partially-swallowed object to completely obstruct the airway.

Some swallowed materials may be aspirated into the lungs and cause spasms of severe coughing. Turning the patient upside down or slapping the individual on the back may push it up into the larynx and if that happens complete obstruction could occur and cause instant death.

So what does the anxious bystander do?

If the victim can't talk and can't take a deep breath and has cyanosis of the lips, then the utmost urgency is demanded. Mouth to mouth resuscitation plus some form of pressure on the upper abdomen as recommended by Heimlich could save the patient's life. It must be remembered, however, that choking spells occur every day and recovery usually takes place spontaneously, except in the most extreme cases.

Eating Meat on Friday

"A patient just arrived in the emergency room. He was eating dinner with family friends and says that a piece of meat is stuck in his throat."

It was the ER supervisor with a very common call on a Friday evening. Usually the complaint was a fish bone that was causing the discomfort.

"Is the patient having any trouble breathing?" I asked almost before she was through speaking.

"No," she said, "but he's gagging a lot and quite uncomfortable."

"Order x-rays of the neck and chest," I said. "Also alert the operating room that I'll probably be doing an esophagoscopy. Since he has food in his stomach I'll be using local anesthesia."

It was shortly after 10 PM when I reached the hospital and checked the patient. Bob was a forty-year-old male who was sitting up on a stretcher retching, but not having any noticeable difficulty in breathing. The x-rays were on the view box and they clearly showed a shadow in the upper esophagus.

The history as given by his wife, Pat, was rather typical of the events frequently leading up to these choking episodes.

"Today is my fortieth birthday and we decided to celebrate the occasion with some of our friends. Suddenly I looked over at Bob who was seated down the row from me. He was gasping for air and pointing to his throat."

The history followed the usual pattern in these choking cases when everybody is having a good time with some over-indulgence in drink and a continuing chatter of voices with everyone talking at the same time.

That's when the catastrophe usually strikes, while the diners are talking, eating, and drinking all at the same time. Some of the food, usually beef as I've already mentioned, is swallowed without proper chewing. The large unchewed piece gets caught in the throat just in back of the windpipe. Other foods such as vegetables will slide down into the stomach, but beef will cause pressure on the airway located immediately in front of the esophagus.

"No one noticed that Bob was having any trouble," Pat continued, "because they were all enjoying themselves. Of course, by then everybody had several drinks, but I never have more than a taste of wine and when I saw Bob gasping I knew he was in trouble. That's when I decided we'd better get him to the hospital as soon as possible. Do you think he'll be alright, Doctor?"

"Bob isn't in any immediate danger," I said, "but the x-rays do show that the piece of steak is caught in the upper part of his esophagus. I'll remove it using local anesthesia and he should be able to go home tomorrow."

After explaining the proposed procedure to Bob and his wife, I went up to the operating room and picked out the instruments for the esophagoscopy. It took but a few more minutes to scrub my hands and put on my gown and when I looked around, my patient hadn't arrived in the room prepared for surgery. I turned to the OR supervisor.

"Please call the ER and find out what's causing the delay," I said. "I'm sure nothing could have happened to my patient since he wasn't having any real difficulty when I left him just a while ago."

In a few minutes she came back with the answer.

"The patient is a Catholic and wants to see the chaplain before going to surgery. Father Hanley is visiting another patient in the hospital and will see him shortly."

My response was immediate and explosive.

"Damn it all," I said, "If he's a Catholic, what the hell's he doing eating meat on Friday?"

This outburst of mine came from a background of strict regimentation in which our family followed the accepted norms of practicing Catholics. Several years later the Vatican Council II changed the church laws that forbade the eating of meat on Friday. This restriction was no different than the tenets of Orthodox Jews and the rigid fundamentalist doctrines of other religions.

Non-Catholics, including most of the Protestant sects, have always been more elastic in their precepts. This has had a lot of appeal to those who sought more freedom in their interpretations of what should guide them in their daily lives.

When my patient finally arrived in the operating room shortly after midnight, the obstructing piece of meat was removed without difficulty. I reassured his wife that he should make an uneventful recovery with no complication from this unfortunate mishap.

The next day, prior to discharge, I gave him the following advice: "Be extra careful to drink alcoholic beverages in moderation, especially when you're eating meat products. Also remember your mother probably taught you never to talk with food in your mouth. It's not the polite thing to do and also dangerous as you have discovered."

I could have suggested that as a Catholic, he might have gone to Hell if he had choked on the meat before arriving at the hospital. But I left that up to the hospital chaplain, Father Hanley. He was a real authoritarian and I'm sure he had reminded my patient of that possibility.

A Catholic Law: No Meat on Friday

"This food has bacon and the church laws say we should not eat it."

This was only one of the statements we heard on that memorable day.

Our local parish had several study groups which met monthly for discussion of the scriptures and their application to family life. It was stimulating and thought-provoking requiring us to spend many hours in preparation for these sessions.

The final event of the year was a social gathering with dinner provided by one of the couples. For this particular summer's evening my wife and I volunteered to be the host and the hostess. Mary was excited about the prospect despite having to spend several days in preparation of a meal that would be appetizing and acceptable to everyone.

Since it was Friday she decided on a dish that observed the obligations of the church, no meat. The mixture containing shrimp, lobster, and scallops had taken hours to put together and my wife was rightfully proud of her concoction.

The guests lined up to fill their plates from the casserole that had been placed on a large drop-leaf table on the porch. Suddenly calamity struck as the first of the group rubbed up against the edge of the table. The drop-leaf dropped with a bang and so did the casserole with all its contents followed by the dishes resting alongside.

Everything crashed to the cement floor of the porch. We had nothing but a mixture of china and the once-delectable seafood. Nothing could be salvaged.

Rather than lend a helping hand to the cleanup job, I took my wife aside and told her I was going to call the pizza shop for a substitute meal.

I could see a look of doubt on my wife's face, but the alternatives were limited. The pizza manager was most cooperative as I outlined our requirements.

"Enough food for sixteen people," I said, "with several different ingredients, but absolutely no meat, do you understand?"

"Sure Doc," he said. "I understand. No meat and enough for sixteen people."

Returning to the group I made my announcement.

"Dinner will be delayed for half an hour and Mary, who is always ready for emergencies, has a surprise dish for you."

I asked the guests to refill their liquid refreshments in the hopes that would diminish their disappointment in the delay of their meal. Soon there was animated conversation again and there was no talk of food.

Right on schedule the pizzas were delivered and I proceeded to uncover each one of them before inviting the hungry couples to dig in. There was only one problem. All the pizzas contained bacon and that was like feeding pork to an orthodox Jew or Muslim.

I turned to our spiritual advisor and asked if there was a theological loophole.

"Under these most unusual and trying circumstances," he intoned, "I will bless this food which we are about to eat."

This instant dispensation relieved us of all guilt and the religious penalty of eating the forbidden fruit. Everyone filled their dishes with the bacon-tainted pizza and nobody developed any swallowing problems. What might have become a disaster turned out to be a fun evening and a conversation piece for a long time afterwards.

Many religions have certain dietary restrictions which they expect their followers to observe. This has been a tradition adopted by the Jews, especially the Orthodox, for thousands of years. Other sects such as the Muslims also forbid the use of pork products by their adherents. Except for the strictly Orthodox, most Jews today don't eliminate pork from their diet nor do they demand kosher food.

Until the Second Vatican Council all Roman Catholics were expected to refrain from the use of meat on Fridays. Being brought up in a strictly religious household, our family observed this edict throughout life until the changes officially took place.

I gave my wife the greatest credit because she remained cool and unflappable during the entire evening, although she did admit to a mild headache the next morning.

Adolph's Meat Tenderizer

"Choking on a piece of meat? Don't worry. There's a simple cure. Use Adolph's Meat Tenderizer."

When this report came out of a small-town newspaper in the south it was quickly published in many other newspapers. The family doctor recommending this approach soon became somewhat of a celebrity for this innovative method.

The use of the tenderizer appeared to be a quick solution for a life-threatening problem.

The rational was based on the fact that this household meat-softener breaks up the tissue fibers of tough meat. The report in the press was followed by several articles in medical journals extolling the use and advantages of this product.

The argument for its use was logical and persuasive. When the tenderizer was taken by teaspoon doses the meat gradually disintegrated, allowing the obstructing bolus of food to become loosened. The piece of meat would then easily pass down into the stomach and no longer be a threat to the patient's life.

The popularity of this treatment was of short duration when it became evident that complications were occurring. Multiple doses of the home treatment resulted in a pooling of the solution around the meat. This caused a breakdown of the esophageal mucosa allowing perforations to occur. Some of the individuals affected developed peritonitis and died. When the reports of fatalities became widely-known, the medical profession strongly advised against the use of Adolph's Meat Tenderizer as a treatment for impacted meat

It's possible that in some areas of the country the treatment is still popular and the choking patient relieved. However, those who try such an approach must be reminded of a well-known axiom, "The cure can sometimes be worse than the disease."

16
Diseases of the Throat

Pharyngitis

The nasopharynx, located at the back of the nose, contains lymphoid tissue called the adenoids. These may grow to large proportions in children causing difficulty in breathing. A more serious complication is right-sided cardiac hypertrophy, a rather rare complication of adenoids that responds to adenoidectomy.

A more common problem from enlarged adenoids is mouth breathing and blockage of the eustachian tube which connects the middle ear to the nasopharynx. This in turn may produce recurrent ear obstruction. If symptoms are severe then adenoidectomy should be considered. This is frequently done without performing a tonsillectomy as had been done routinely in the past.

The pharynx, which starts at the back of the mouth, carries air from the nose to the lungs. It also carries food from the mouth to the esophagus.

Tonsillitis is the most common infection of the pharynx and these knobs of lymphoid tissue located on each side of the throat have been the most common object of surgery until recent years. The introduction of antibiotics has reduced the need for tonsillectomy. However, repeated attacks of infection and resistance to medical treatment are two conditions that will continue to demand tonsil surgery, especially if the patient's symptoms cause increased loss of school attendance and absence from the work force in the older adult.

Complications of tonsillectomy are primarily due to bleeding that can occur when a blood vessel erupts several hours and occasionally as long as up to five to seven days after surgery. This is a problem that can happen after any operative procedure, but is readily controlled by the trained surgeon.

Pharyngitis, acute and chronic, is one of the more common causes of time lost from school and work. The sore throat experienced may also be related to a postnasal drip, exposure to a dry environment especially in the winter season, and very importantly, excessive smoking and overuse of alcohol.

Treatment of the acute painful discomfort includes gargling with warm water and Karo syrup or anesthetic lozenges such as aspergum. When the secretion is thick and greenish it indicates a possible secondary infection. A culture may reveal a bug that can be controlled by an antibiotic. The persistent recurrent chronic pharyngitis often responds to the daily use of a nasal douche containing eight ounces of warm water and one-half teaspoon of salt. Even more effective is a douche of equal parts of Alkalol and water.

Laryngitis, or hoarseness as it's commonly called, can be a minor temporary problem or a precursor of a life-threatening disease.

Acute laryngitis is usually brought on by an upper respiratory infection, vocal abuse such as screaming at some gatherings such as sporting events, talking too much, or an unusual amount of smoking or drinking at a social affair. Treatment requires no more than voice rest and steam inhalations two or three times a day until the voice returns to normal. Antihistamines aren't advised since they worsen the condition by increasing the dryness of the vocal cords.

Chronic laryngitis lasting more than two weeks can be caused by a number of factors any one of which demands attention by a physician, preferably an ENT specialist. The hoarseness may be due to a benign growth or a malignant tumor, but sometimes it may be due to a paralyzed vocal cord caused by an injury to the laryngeal nerve in the neck. It might be the first sign of a serious disease involving the brain or even a metastatic tumor from some other organ.

Benign vocal cord growths are small nodules diagnosed with a laryngeal mirror examination, but often a correct diagnosis may require a direct laryngoscopy under anesthesia. Treatment is excision, preferably with the aid of the microscope. Examination by the pathologist will confirm whether the tumor is benign or malignant.

Malignant vocal cord growths are usually suspected of their deadly nature when the patient is first seen by the throat specialist. Final diagnosis, of course, is determined by the pathologist. If definitely malignant, immediate treatment is necessary.

The specific treatment depends on the type and location of the tumor. If the tumor is discovered early, then radiation or removal of the affected cord will allow preservation of the larynx, an acceptable voice, and almost a 100% chance of a cure. It is one of the most curable cancers when the patient sees the throat specialist in the early stages of his hoarseness.

Psychogenic Loss of Voice

The mother of thirteen-year-old Louise gave a short history after she was referred from the pediatrician.

"Louise has been healthy most of her life," she said. "Two months ago she awoke and could barely speak above a whisper. Later in the day she regained her normal speaking voice so I canceled the appointment I made with her doctor."

"What happened after that?" I said.

"A month ago she started to whisper again and this time her speech continued that way. The family and her friends couldn't understand her. After a week I decided this time she should be seen by the pediatrician. He put her on a throat spray and prescribed some pills, but nothing seems to help. Now she doesn't want to go to school because she can't talk in class or to her friends."

I asked Louise a few simple questions and got a whispered response. I sprayed her throat with a light anesthetic. She was a most cooperative patient. By using the laryngeal mirror I saw the vocal cords clearly and they were perfectly normal.

I was baffled for a while as to what treatment I could prescribe to bring back her speech since there wasn't anything wrong with her vocal cords that I could see. Then I recalled several months earlier a meeting held in Boston where one of the speakers described several cases of patients with a sudden loss of voice. Dr. Beck attributed the problem to hysteria and in each case he encouraged the patient to speak normally. After this failed to bring any improvement he decided to use another approach.

"When coaxing failed to produce normal speech I used a little subterfuge which at that time I called pseudo-psychology."

This fatherly physician from upstate New York described what proved to be an effective approach for his patients.

"Without spraying the throat," he said, "I took a long cotton-tipped wire probe and told the patient that this was going to bring her voice back to normal. I pushed the probe deep into the throat until she developed severe noisy gagging. I then told the patients they could now start talking normally again and they all did."

In the case of Louise I figured nothing ventured, nothing gained. With her mother sitting close by, the patient was told that my treatment was going to bring back her speech, but she might feel a little uncomfortable with the procedure.

Following the approach used by Dr. Beck, I inserted the long cotton-tipped wire probe deep into her throat. Louise coughed and gagged so severely I thought she was going to vomit. I then withdrew the probe and told her to repeat after me, "One, two, three..." She did well until she reached six, when once again her voice went off into a whisper. I was baffled again momentarily, but I quickly decided on a solution.

"Louise, you have two vocal cords, but I only touched one. Now we are going to do the same thing to the other cord."

The young lady readily agreed to my suggestion. Her ready acceptance convinced me she really wanted to talk and only needed some positive encouragement.

The same procedure was repeated with the gagging reaction following which the patient began to count and stopped at ten as I had requested. I then told Louise she was cured and would need no further treatment. She smiled and began to talk to her mother cheerfully and almost nonstop. Her response was much more dramatic and complete than I anticipated.

Frankly, I felt somewhat like a charlatan by resorting to such deception in telling her my treatment was going to bring back her speech. Actually it was the power of suggestion that produced the result. That is true in so many situations we face in life, not just in the practice of medicine.

From my initial examination I knew Louise had no disease of the vocal cords and therefore it had to be a psychologically-induced problem.

Louise sat in the waiting room while I talked with her mother and explained the problem to her. I told her I had no idea why it had developed. She told me Louise had begun her menses just before the speech loss first took place. Her voice had returned to normal at that time, but the recurrence of her symptoms developed with the onset of her menstrual flow the following month, but this time the speech loss persisted. I'm sure this was the precipitating factor in her failure to speak, but I had no explanation for the persistence of her symptoms following the second monthly period. I did suggest to the pediatrician that a recurrence of her problem would demand a psychological evaluation. I heard nothing further from her doctor and I presumed my diagnosis and treatment were correct.

17
Cancer

Cancer of the Larynx

"Cancer of the larynx has one of the highest rates of curability if it's diagnosed early."

Based on my experience and that of many others, this is a statement that cannot be easily refuted. However, when the word cancer is mentioned it spreads terror into the mind and heart of almost everyone. This fear is understandable since so many cancers can be fatal, despite every attempt to control the disease. Unfortunately, many individuals delay seeking medical attention because of their dread of cancer. All too frequently a malignancy with a high degree of curability is allowed to progress beyond the point where a life or even an involved organ might be saved.

One of the most satisfying rewards in medicine for me was to see a patient early in the stages of a malignancy involving the larynx. At that point it would be almost possible to guarantee a cure of the disease with only minimal effect on speech.

Most of us have at sometime or other experienced a distortion of the voice such as hoarseness or laryngitis. Invariably this is associated with a cold or abuse of the voice. The two vocal cords which meet in the larynx and vibrate to create the sound are very fragile and easily irritated. When this happens the voice undergoes changes. Voice rest usually promotes a return to normal speech and no other treatment is needed. However, if the infection or overuse and abuse persist then the hoarseness will continue and frequently become more severe.

The most difficult patient a physician encounters is the one who smokes or drinks to excess. This is especially true if both of these habits are present and this, unfortunately, is very common. How often do we attend social affairs and observe the guests holding a cigarette in one hand and a drink in the other. A mathematical formula could be easily established stating that T (tobacco) plus A (alcohol) equals C (cancer). Such an equation isn't absolute, but after years in practice I found it was all too frequently true.

When the symptoms of hoarseness last more than two weeks, it's almost imperative that the patient be evaluated by a throat specialist. For the patient who constantly abuses his larynx, especially with tobacco and alcohol, evaluation of the hoarseness should not be delayed beyond two weeks.

Smoking and Cancer

"If you're going to smoke, get your chest x-rays every six months so we can diagnose and treat your cancer early."

These words were spoken by Dr. Alton Ochsner at an ENT meeting I attended in New Orleans in the 1950s. Dr. Ochsner, a world-famous chest surgeon, was one of the first believers in the relationship of cigarette smoking to cancer of the lung.

As he gave his talk, clouds of smoke enshrouded the assembly hall. The message at that time hadn't gotten through to the throat specialists, but Ochsner's remarks were foreboding.

For many years at the national meetings of the Academy of Otolaryngology, Camel cigarettes had one of the busiest booths in the convention hall. Doctors were lined up to receive their free package of cigarettes. The Camel manufacturers had a clever public relations department then and they still do.

Stimulated by the published scientific articles as well as the stand taken by the leading members of the ENT societies, it appeared to me some forceful action was needed. After consulting with the chest physicians and the ENT department, I presented a motion at the monthly meeting of the hospital staff.

"In view of the relationship of smoking to cancer of the lung and emphysema, it is recommended that the ladies auxiliary remove all cigarette machines from the hospital areas."

The hospital staff turned down the motion despite the knowledge of reports showing the relationship of lung cancer to the use of tobacco. At this time a large percentage of physicians were heavy smokers. Being so-called rugged individualists, they resented any interference with access to purchase tobacco products.

My efforts weren't wasted since word of my proposal reached the members of the ladies auxiliary executive committee. Although the auxiliary contributed many thousands of dollars through the sale of these cigarettes, they agreed to remove the dispensing machines from the hospital areas. Word of their action spread to other area hospitals and eventually the proposal was adopted by all other medical facilities in the state.

How to Quit Smoking

"Why did you quit smoking?"

The patient was a forty-year-old male who was being seen for the first time because of a mild hearing loss caused by the accumulation of wax. Whenever a patient was examined for any ENT complaint, I included a question about smoking habits.

This gentleman went on to say he had smoked two packs a day for almost twenty years. While attending a social event he reached into his pocket for a cigarette and then realized he already had one in his mouth.

"At that moment I decided I was hooked. I took the cigarette out of my mouth and threw it away. Then I tossed the half-empty package into a wastebasket."

"How long ago was that?"

"That was three years ago and I still have a desire for a cigarette, but now that feeling quickly passes."

Such a dramatic cessation is unusual since most smokers have severe withdrawal symptoms and quitting is not easy. For the addicted smoker it amounts to torture while struggling to give up the habit.

A friend of mine was a two-pack-a-day smoker and during a social evening he could be seen lighting up one cigarette after another. Because of our close friendship there wasn't any hesitancy on my part in being a little forceful.

"Bill," I said to him one day, "you can't keep up this filthy habit without affecting your lungs. Quit while you're ahead."

"Doc, I feel fine and smoking is one of the few pleasures I truly enjoy."

Several months later when I saw him he greeted me with a broad smile.

"I was just checked by my doctor three weeks ago and he showed me the chest film. The x-ray showed the beginning of emphysema and he insisted that I stop smoking immediately."

This middle-aged gentleman has now gone four years without smoking, but he admits he hasn't lost the desire for a cigarette.

Some years ago I met a former neighbor at a local shopping mall. He was accompanied by his wife as he carried a small oxygen tank for breathing. We chatted for a few minutes and then he recalled a visit to my office a few years earlier.

"You might not remember, Doctor, but I saw you for a sore throat. You told me then I should quit my two-pack-a-day cigarette habit. If I had listened to you at that time, I probably wouldn't be lugging this machine around the past three years."

Two years later I learned this fifty-year-old man had passed away after being hospitalized with severe breathing difficulties.

It is doubly disturbing to hear such patients had succumbed to the effects of tobacco addiction. First, my words of caution weren't sufficient to influence a decision to give up smoking. Secondly, I became a predictor of a fatal ending and there isn't any satisfaction in realizing the truth of my caution.

There are many highly-advertised approaches that claim success in stopping the addiction to smoking. The cures range from acupuncture to vitamin Z. For several years the nicotine patch enjoyed popularity. This too has lost some of its attractiveness and has now been replaced by a so-called double-strength patch.

Psychotherapy, transcendental meditation, smoke-enders, and a multitude of other groups and individuals lay claim to successful results in terminating smoking. As with weight loss ventures the vast majority of these individuals fail to maintain their initial encouraging objectives.

The patient who is faced with an "either or" prediction by his or her physician is the one most likely to take the steps necessary to be a winner in the race for a tobacco-free life. Failure to heed the danger signs or adopting the attitude "Well, I have to die from something," will end up in disaster.

The tobacco industry has done a very successful job in starting young people in a habit that is totally addictive despite the lowering of the nicotine content and the use of filters. The billions of dollars poured into advertising and the support of political office holders will continue to frustrate the efforts of health providers who seek legislation to curb the use of tobacco.

Several centuries ago Great Britain became alarmed at the rapid rise of alcoholism. A huge tax on alcohol lowered the intake of whiskey and the death rate from alcoholism. Taxing each pack of cigarettes with a $5.00 stamp would bring about a dramatic drop in cigarette sales, especially among teenagers. Don't look for such a tax in the next millennium. The tobacco industry doesn't want it and the politicians are not about to bite the hand that feeds them.

Mickey's Cancer Surgery

"Has my patient arrived yet?" I asked the ward nurse who answered the phone.

"Not yet," she replied.

I couldn't understand what might have happened to Mickey

O'Connell, a sixty-year-old white male whom I admitted to the hospital two days earlier. He had a history of hoarseness for almost one year when I first saw him in the office a week before. After the examination I told him he had a growth on his vocal cord that looked very much like a cancer, but luckily it was located in an area that had a good chance of being cured if treated immediately. With some understandable hesitation, he finally agreed to hospitalization for a biopsy of the lesion.

There wasn't any question at the Friday morning biopsy surgery that this was a malignant growth. However, before telling Mickey of my own feelings I told him we would await the pathologist's report the following day. After all, the surgeon can be quite sure of his own judgement in such cases, but on occasion the report turns out to be negative.

The next morning I checked the slides with the pathologist and my suspicions were confirmed that Mickey did have a cancer. At the time of the surgical biopsy I was able to determine this growth could be removed with only the loss of one vocal cord. With such a procedure a hoarse-speaking voice would occur, but this is a minor problem compared to the complete removal of the larynx. In many cases the cancer has already spread to both sides of the larynx and beyond, thus necessitating the removal of the entire voice box unless radiation therapy is chosen instead of surgery.

When I talked with Mickey shortly afterwards and explained what had to be done, he was surprisingly receptive. He was happy to know he would still be able to speak adequately despite the planned surgery.

I believed that I had pretty well prepared him for the diagnosis, but after our discussion Mickey had one request.

"Dr. Curran, you're planning to operate on Monday, right?"

"That's right, Mickey," I replied.

"Well, why should I stay here all day today and tomorrow, sitting around doing nothing except worrying? Why can't I leave here now and come back tonight? My niece is getting married this afternoon and I really want to go to the wedding. I'll be back here tonight after the reception and be ready for the operation on Monday morning."

After making a weak effort to convince Mickey that hospital regulations didn't allow such arrangements, I agreed to recommend the pass that would permit him to leave the hospital and re-occupy his room later in the day. Mickey took off shortly afterwards in a very happy mood and he promised to return that evening about 6 PM.

I called the nurse at that time to make sure that he had arrived. They had not seen or heard from my patient. Being rather concerned I called again at 8 o'clock and again at 10 o'clock, but there was no sign of

Mickey. I asked the nurse to call me if and when he returned.

It was 1 AM when a call came from my answering service asking me to contact the hospital floor where Mickey was located. The first question I asked the nurse was, "Did Mickey O'Connell check in?"

"He did not check in," she replied. "He rolled in."

In retrospect my next question was rather dumb, I must admit.

"How is Mickey feeling?"

Her reply was instantaneous. "He's feeling no pain," she said.

Mickey definitely needed no medication to help him sleep that night. He did admit to a hangover headache the next morning. He also thanked me for allowing him to have the time out of the hospital to attend the wedding.

The surgery on Monday morning went off without any complications and he was discharged a week later.

I followed Mickey for some years after his successful surgery, and he never failed to remind me that it was the best wedding reception he had ever attended.

Perseverance Wins a Cancer Battle

"Hello, Dr. Curran. How are you today?"

When John Gilmore greeted me with a clear esophageal voice, I knew his battle had been won.

This fifty-year-old black man was one of my early cases of laryngeal cancer. As John spoke I recalled his examination many months earlier when I first saw him with a history of hoarseness.

"How long has your voice been like this?" I had asked him before looking at his throat.

"About two months," he said, "but nothing seems to help. The druggist gave me some lozenges and then I saw my family doctor and he prescribed some expensive antibiotics, but those didn't help either."

When seeing a patient with hoarseness, I never ask them if they smoke or drink. I put the question more directly.

"How much do you smoke, John?"

"Two packs a day," he answered quickly, "but I don't inhale."

That is a stock answer for most smokers.

"How much do you drink?"

"I spend a few hours a night with my friends at our neighborhood bar, but only on weekends and I never have more than a couple of beers."

A "couple" could be somewhere between two and six.

Examination of the patient's larynx showed some thick whitish spots on both vocal cords. These had the typical appearance of a condition known as leukoplakia. Dentists often see such a tissue change in the patient's mouth and will usually biopsy the area involved since often there may be malignant changes requiring further surgery or treatment.

I explained this to the patient.

"John, you have some suspicious areas on your vocal cords that have to be checked. I'll admit you to the hospital for a minor operation to examine the area more closely under anesthesia. At the same time some of that tissue will be removed for examination by the pathologist."

The biopsy report confirmed my suspicions of leukoplakia, but in the opinion of the pathologist there were no malignant cells.

John was most cooperative and understanding when I outlined what precautions he should take to minimize the possibility of cancer cells developing. Since he was a gregarious man who wanted to continue enjoying an occasional evening with his friends, I knew my suggestions might not be readily acceptable. Sitting with his friends in a smoke-filled room enjoying a few drinks was certainly more enjoyable than spending those hours at home worrying about the possibility of a cancer developing. However, he did agree to quit smoking and limit his beer intake to two glasses.

I arranged to have John checked at my office every month so that I would have a chance to gauge his progress. Any changes in his speech would be readily noted by him, but more importantly, I wanted to know if the vocal cords had changed in appearance in any way.

Although his voice did improve I noted that one cord looked some-what irregular on his third monthly visit to the office. John agreed to a hospital admission for another biopsy. This time the pathologist's report wasn't good. There were cancer cells present on one of the vocal cords. A biopsy of the opposite cord showed some thickening but no cancer.

I was now faced with a real dilemma. Should the cancerous cord be removed or would radiation cure the malignancy and prevent cancer from developing on the opposite cord? After consulting with the radi-ologists and my ENT colleagues, I decided radiation was the more ac-ceptable approach.

My patient agreed readily when the reason for the treatment was thoroughly explained to him.

"I hope we can avoid any surgery involving the removal of the vo-cal cords," I said. "The treatment will require six weeks of daily radia-tion, but it won't cause any discomfort."

During the early weeks of treatment, John was noticeably depressed. Although I tried to assume an air of optimism and satisfaction with his progress, it was impossible to promise a cure. When the radiation was completed and his voice improved, he became more cheerful.

For the next three months John was checked on a weekly basis. Each time he greeted me with a smile that seemed to broaden after each examination.

"The vocal cords look good," I said, "and we might have a cure, but I'll have to check you regularly for a few more months. And don't forget, no smoking."

The fourth month following his radiation I noted some suspicious changes in both vocal cords. At this time the patient noticed increased hoarseness which was my own observation, also.

John's pleasant smile vanished after I finished my examination of the larynx.

"You have a few spots on your cords that don't look good. These will have to be biopsied. Let's wait until we get the report before we decide what has to be done."

"If the report shows cancer, Dr. Curran, will that mean my voice box will have to be removed?"

"Probably so, John, since you have already had a course of radiation. But let's see what the biopsy tells us."

Under anesthesia the cords were more completely visualized with the laryngoscope and there was little doubt as to the diagnosis. The tissues showed marked irregularities on both sides and the biopsies were reported by the pathologist as cancer on both sides of the larynx.

When I walked into his room the next day, I think my patient had a premonition of the diagnosis.

"John, I'm sorry to say the tissue removed from both cords shows cancer"

There was no hesitation as he immediately asked, "When are you going to operate, Doctor?"

From the beginning of his first treatment, the alternative approaches had been discussed with the patient. The pros and cons of radiation and surgery were outlined so there would be no question as to why each step was taken. Now the reason for the surgery and the problems involved in recovering from such a procedure were fully explained. The loss of the larynx can be a terrifying situation to the patients who believe that it will render them mute.

"When the larynx is removed, John, there are several ways you can carry on a conversation with your family and friends. You can learn what we call esophageal speech, and if necessary, an electro-larynx can be used."

My explanation seemed to encourage John. I was amazed at his eagerness to accept the challenge and get on with the operation. The total laryngectomy was performed and in less than two weeks, John was discharged from the hospital.

My patient's attitude was outstanding and I complimented him on his courage.

"John, you amaze me the way you have accepted this surgical procedure. It's not easy to go through all the frustrations you have experienced and not lose hope. I'm proud of you. Now let's get started on your speech therapy."

John Gilmore's efforts to develop esophageal speech after surgery were unsuccessful. Try as he might, he was unable to get the words to come out. I contacted a speech therapist, who had some limited experience in teaching laryngectomized patients how to develop a speaking voice. This also ended in failure.

Since John was becoming more discouraged and depressed, I arranged for him to obtain an electro-larynx. This artificial larynx served two purposes. It allowed John to communicate with his family and friends and that raised his spirits. It also gave him enough incentive to pursue his efforts to develop esophageal speech which he wanted to acquire. The monotone response with the electronic gadget was not very satisfying to him.

He came to the office one day for his weekly visit and complained about it.

"Doctor, I don't like using this damn thing," he said, "but when I swallow air (esophageal speech) I can't seem to get my words out and I sound terrible. I just don't know what to do. I'm really discouraged."

For over a month John failed to keep his regular appointments and I was concerned that he might be developing a recurrence of his disease or some other unexpected complication. About five weeks after his last visit, John walked into my office and greeted me in a distinctly-sounding esophageal voice.

"Hello, Dr. Curran. How are you?"

As he sat in my office his words flowed out without difficulty and with complete clarity. There was no need to ask him how it all happened. With no prompting from me, he proceeded to give me a full accounting of what had occurred.

"My wife isn't a nagging person, but she occasionally became impatient and annoyed when she couldn't understand what I was trying to say. One day, while she was off to work, I decided that something had to be done."

I listened intently but said nothing as he carried on his esophageal speech without hesitation, not even stopping to catch his breath. Swallowing air and using the throat and chest muscles to help form the words in the mouth can be tiring, but John was like a long-distance runner who wanted to reach the finish line.

He continued to explain what had happened.

"I sat down on the side of the bed and convinced myself I was going to learn to talk. I kept at it until I became exhausted, but I didn't give up. Finally everything began to come through clearly. When my wife came home that night I don't know which one of us was happier."

The desperate extra effort was all John needed. He didn't require any further encouragement from me to become once again the affable, sociable person he had always been. On his later visits to my office he would delight me by describing his activities since his previous checkup. He always enjoyed going to church, but since he couldn't communicate as he wished, he had avoided attending services. Now he was once again part of the congregation. He loved to dance and this again was a social event he and his wife could now enjoy.

Patients undergoing total laryngectomy need some encouragement that all will not be lost when the larynx is removed. I decided to ask John for some help.

"John, as you already know, losing your voice box can be pretty scary. Would you be willing to see some of these patients before and after surgery so they can be encouraged about being able to speak again?

"Dr. Curran, I owe my life to you. I'll be glad to do anything that can help them realize they can talk as well as I do."

John Gilmore never hesitated to visit these patients in the hospital during the several days before the surgery as well as postoperatively. Where so many were overcome with despair, John brought them hope as he displayed his ability to speak. When asked to give talks to medical groups and civic organizations I could always depend upon John to tell the audience how he overcame the loss of his larynx. He did it in an entertaining manner so the listeners were captivated by his frank and truly dramatic presentation.

On several occasions when I was asked to discuss laryngeal cancer on radio or television, I called on John to join me and demonstrate his ability to communicate.

Prior to our first TV appearance, John was somewhat apprehensive.

"I'm afraid I'll be nervous and won't know what to say."

"You will do and talk exactly as you have been doing when we speak before groups of doctors, nurses, and various civic groups."

In such presentations I always asked him what his first reactions were to the diagnosis of cancer and the loss of his larynx. Following his responses I would lead him on to discuss his eventual success in developing a good esophageal speech.

As soon as we started our presentation on TV, John began to talk. I became part of the supporting cast and he became the star of the show.

John lived some twenty years after his laryngectomy. He survived gallbladder surgery, a heart attack, and multiple other ailments, but after each recovery he continued to give talks whenever the occasion arose.

By encouraging the victims of throat cancer to face their disease he implanted a strong seed of hope where there might have been despair. He was truly a doctor's assistant without any medical training but a strong desire to help his fellow man. I know there are many people like John in this world, but I was lucky to have him as a patient and as a friend. He made my life as a physician much more fulfilling and for that I am forever grateful.

Unusual Neck Swelling
A Near Fatality

"Doctor, the pharmacist at Netherlands Drug Store just called. A man is there holding a slip of paper with your name on it and he's having trouble breathing."

As soon as my secretary gave me the message I knew the person in distress had to be Jim Boudreau. A month earlier a man in his 50s was referred to me by another physician. The patient had a swelling on the left side of his neck. This enlarged area caused him no symptoms but he said it was gradually increasing in size over a period of several months. X-rays confirmed my suspicion that he had a cyst of the larynx, called a laryngocele. This relatively rare condition is basically an anomalous air sac that is connected to the larynx . It produces a tumor-like lesion on the side of the neck but this case was also noted to contain fluid and is diagnosed as a pyolaryngocele which means that there is infection in the cyst.

Surgery was advised since an infection in such cysts had been reported to cause difficulty in breathing and occasionally ended fatally. The patient failed to appear for his admission to the hospital and couldn't be reached at his home by phone. His place of employment was also contacted and I found out he hadn't worked since his visit to my office.

A letter was sent to the patient alerting him again to the dangers that might occur if surgery was postponed. Three weeks went by with no response. My worst fears were realized that afternoon when my secretary burst into the treatment room with that telephone call while I was examining a patient.

I grabbed a sharp-pointed surgical knife from the instrument drawer

and raced down to the drugstore a few hundred feet away. As I anticipated, it was Jim Boudreau who was gasping, unable to talk, and having
great difficulty breathing. I decided to forego emergency surgery in the
drugstore since there wasn't any evidence of severe obstruction to his
air passages except for some bluish discoloration of his lips.

A physician friend, Dr. Duffy, who was in the drugstore at the time,
offered to drive the patient and me to the hospital less than a mile away.
While making a U-turn against the oncoming traffic we were stopped
by a patrol officer. One look at the gasping patient cradled in my arms
required no explanation to the policeman. He jumped into his car, turned
on his flashing red lights and siren and led us to the hospital emergency
room within a matter of minutes.

The patient was wheeled up to the operating room immediately after he arrived in the emergency room. In that short period of time his
breathing had become much worse. His chest muscles were retracting
severely as he gasped almost convulsively for air. His entire face was
now turning to a bluish discoloration. I wondered if I had hesitated too
long by not doing the tracheotomy at the drugstore.

Once we were in the operating suite and without changing into a
scrub suite, I grasped the knife from the outstretched hand of the nurse,
who recognized immediately what was happening and I quickly made
the incision in the patient's neck for the tracheotomy. There was instant
relief of the patient's labored breathing as a blast of air came flowing
through the neck opening. The patient's color quickly turned to pink as
he breathed easier. I breathed easier, too, as a sense of relaxation came
over me now that the tensions of the previous few minutes were over.

Two days later I excised the cyst successfully without any complications. The pathologist identified it as a pyolaryngocele as was suspected by the x-rays as well as the breathing difficulty that had developed. The patient made a full recovery and was discharged from the
hospital within a week.

Why had Jim Boudreau failed to return for his surgery as I had
requested?

Following recovery from his surgery he told me the whole story. He
and his wife were separated after she discovered he was keeping company with another woman. She was infuriated. She sued him for support
and a subpoena had been issued for him to appear in court which he was
trying to avoid. It almost cost him his life.

I never learned of the outcome of the legal battle that was about to
erupt between Jim Boudreau and his wife since there wasn't any request
for me to testify. From the medical standpoint, however, I was happy
my patient survived.

18
Malpractice

Winning a Malpractice Suit

"We represent the interests of our client who was examined by your audiologist. During the test the left ear was injured and his neck was twisted, requiring medical treatment. Please notify your insurance carrier."

When I received this letter from the attorney, I was stunned and emotionally disturbed. I picked up the phone and called the office of the plaintiff's attorney. He wasn't available so I left a message.

"I'm going to fight the case," I said, "and after I win my action I intend countersuing for malicious and purposeless conduct."

I should have saved my breath and my time. In the State of Connecticut I learned later, a physician is not allowed to countersue an attorney. The legislature, which is controlled by attorneys, had decreed that the plaintiff has a right to seek redress and it's the attorney's responsibility to support his plea.

A recent issue of the Reader's Digest pointed out that the most powerful lobby in Washington and the United States is the American Trial Lawyers Association.

After venting my frustration and anger with my call to the plaintiff's lawyer, I called my insurance agent. He notified the insurance company's legal counsel, who responded very quickly. He strongly advised against any communication with the plaintiff or his attorneys. I told him nothing about my outburst.

When the insurance lawyer visited me at my office for a deposition I had a sense he wanted a quick settlement.

I categorically denied there was any fault associated with my care or that of my audiologist and furthermore, I wasn't interested in any settlement. Several months later I received a list of complaints submitted by the patient's attorney. I realized then why the docket was crowded with suits of all kinds and why the insurance company was anxious to settle as soon as possible.

In reviewing my records I noted the patient had been seen by me following referral from a manufacturing company in the area. He stated he had developed a hearing loss from his exposure to noise at his job at the factory. Testing reports at his workplace showed the noise level, which was slightly above normal, wouldn't produce the loss claimed by the worker.

At the time of my initial examination, the patient gave a history of a buzzing (tinnitus) in the ears which, according to the pre-employment records, had existed for some time before he worked at the factory. Following my evaluation I referred the patient to our hearing center audiologist. His report confirmed my impression. The patient's hearing loss was most likely related to hereditary factors, but not due to noise exposure at his work.

During my years of practice I had occasion to examine many patients who developed varying degrees of deafness secondary to loud sounds either from employment or accidental exposure. Such hearing losses are and should be compensable.

Early in my years as an ENT specialist, I realized the need to employ an audiologist who was trained to use the most modern techniques in evaluating a patient's hearing loss. This enabled me not only to treat the patient more efficiently, but also to help establish the correct diagnosis and cause of the deafness. It was an inherent protection for the patient as well as the employer.

I could understand why the patient wasn't happy with my original report, but based on my examination and the audiologist's evaluation, I had no alternative except to state his hearing loss wasn't caused by his work environment.

As the years went by I certainly didn't expect to hear anything further, so it came as a complete surprise to receive a request from the Workman's Compensation commission for a reexamination of this same patient. The worker was approaching retirement age and apparently still felt he had a case for some monetary compensation.

At this time I repeated my examination and followed it up with another complete testing by the audiologist. The results were substantially the same although there was a slight worsening of the hearing as was to be expected. Advancing age will cause further loss of hearing because of the circulatory changes that take place in the inner ear.

When these evaluations were finished I thought the whole case was put to rest. It was a total surprise to receive the notification from the patient's attorney about two years after my last evaluation. It was claimed that damage to the patient's ear and neck occurred during the audiometric testing.

The claim representative for the insurance company wasn't much help. She questioned the fact that my audiologist was an employee and not an independent contractor. This would make the insurance company not liable for his actions and therefore not covered by my malpractice policy. My audiologist, Paul, would therefore be personally liable.

I was able to prove by my payroll sheets that he was indeed an employee and therefore covered by my policy. I was then advised there was a $100,000 limit on my policy and any jury settlement beyond that was my personal responsibility.

I swallowed hard on the claim agent's contention and suggestions, but I wasn't about to give in and make a settlement. It made me wonder who was working for whom, but I realized the insurance company just wanted to get rid of these cases as soon as possible and avoid any extensive litigation which could prove costly. No wonder our premiums are so high.

In a further attempt to censure my audiologist for his evaluation, the plaintiff's attorney accused him of failing to keep his testing equipment in proper order. We rechecked the records and the equipment knowing we could refute this claim. However, I could see this was one lawyer who was going to pull out all stops in order to get a hefty settlement. After reviewing this whole case, I became more convinced than ever about the total lack of justification for the legal action being taken.

Before hiring Paul as an audiologist, I had checked his credentials and learned he had a degree in audiology from the University of Connecticut. He was also in the process of earning credits for a Ph.D in audiology. He had been working part-time at the medical school in their audiology department and was given nothing but the highest of recommendations by his supervisors.

In the beginning I also observed him as he tested the patients. He was kind, considerate, and interested in their hearing difficulties. Patients on their return to my office would often comment on his pleasant, affable, and efficient manner.

I was therefore particularly incensed when the bill of particulars presented by the plaintiff's attorney implied Paul had not used proper technique and knowledge. It stated when the audiologist turned up the volume for testing his client the intensity was so severe it caused the patient's ears to ring and this problem had since persisted. It also claimed that during my audiologist's attempts to adjust the testing phones on the ears he had twisted the patient's neck so severely that neck spasms developed requiring treatment by his family doctor for over a year since the examination was done.

If I hadn't been cautioned by my attorney I'm sure I would have picked up the phone and really blasted the plaintiff's lawyer for this obvious falsehood. I also wanted to question the honesty, ability, and integrity of the family doctor who had been giving the neck therapy.

I restrained my emotions and called the audiologist over to my office and explained what had taken place. He was concerned and also somewhat alarmed at the prospect of being involved in any action which might question his competence and integrity as well as any financial liability to which he might be subject.

I reassured him his only involvement was to produce the records of the examination with his interpretation. As his employer I was financially responsible for his actions in any suit being brought. Although he was still disturbed by the case he was relieved he wasn't going to be burdened by any monetary loss.

Over the following two years I called my insurance company attorney at regular intervals to see what progress was being made. I did insist from the very beginning that I would refuse to approve any settlement. This was pigheadedness on my part, but I did have a sense of professional pride and knew that neither I nor my audiologist had been guilty of any negligence in the care and evaluation of this patient.

I realized that not infrequently suits are brought up by some lawyers without any justification. They are aware of the fact that insurance companies will pay off the claimant to avoid litigation which could be costly if prolonged. I refused to go along with this nuisance-type agreement and I emphasized this whenever I spoke to my attorney. Again I know this was a stupid reaction, but after being in practice for forty years without any action ever being taken against me I wanted to go out with a clean slate.

My lawyer was encouraging by his observation the plaintiff's attorney was having trouble getting the services of any professionally-trained audiologist who was willing to testify my employee, Paul, had been negligent in any way. In addition we were able to line up several audiologists from the university who would vouch for Paul.

As the months went by I became a little anxious since I had decided on the date of my retirement and I wanted no loose strings hanging on after the date of my departure. However, the retirement date came without any progress.

I closed my office for good and turned my compass southward to Florida for the winter. Following my departure I received a note from my attorney that the opposing counsel was still trying to line up some expert witnesses but was unsuccessful.

My lawyer also advised the clerk of the court I was now residing in Florida and wouldn't be returning for six to eight months. I heard no more of the case during my absence and figured no news was good news. I called my attorney when I returned in June and asked if the suit had been dropped. No such luck. The action was on the court docket awaiting the plaintiff's next move.

A month later on July 15, I had a call from my lawyer. The trial was set for the next day. I told him "no way." I had made plans to go to Vermont for three days with some friends and I didn't intend to break the arrangements. I did have some apprehension during those three days that I might have to face not a day or a week, but possibly a month or more trying to defend myself against a cooked-up complaint. I called the attorney on my return from Vermont and asked him what had happened. It was good news. The entire action had been dropped.

I was naturally curious as to what had taken place after all these years without any developments. I was amazed when my attorney described the steps leading to the cancellation of the suit.

The plaintiff's attorney approached my counsel at the courthouse and offered to settle for $10,000. My lawyer respecting my wishes refused the offer. The demands then dropped to $5,000 then $1,000, all of which were refused.

The payoff was when the lawyer asked if a settlement of $500 would be made to cover his expenses. This approach was made despite the fact that all this time my attorney was reminding the plaintiff's legal counsel I wouldn't agree to pay one dime.

When the last request for payment was also turned down the case was withdrawn and finally closed. That also brought to a finish one of the most exasperating episodes in my life as a physician. I'm not sure I acted smartly in refusing to make a settlement in the beginning. It could have ended disastrously for me as has happened to so many of my colleagues.

Sometime after my case was closed I read a story in the New York Times about a physician who advised a patient his symptoms of chest pain indicated a possible heart problem and recommended hospitalization. The patient refused the suggestion since he claimed he had certain obligations he wished to fulfill. The next day he suffered a severe heart attack.

According to the news report the patient instituted a suit against the doctor because he failed to insist upon hospitalization. The case dragged on for a year at the end of which time the seventy-two-year-old male physician took his own life.

Over the years I have had a number of articles relating to medical experiences that were published in assorted medical journals. These were joyful happenings in most cases, but occasionally were traumatic.

One of my published articles described the agony I suffered with my lung cancer scare. My description of this threatening episode in my life was not only accepted for publication, but put me in the running for the grand prize, a trip to Hawaii. I lost out to a radiologist who successfully countersued a plaintiff's attorney who had sued him for malpractice.

The x-ray specialist not only won his case, but also obtained a judgement against the attorney for the false claims made against him. This happened in Illinois, one of the few states where a countersuit can be instituted. The radiologist certainly deserved his reward. I know it was pride in my work and my employees that motivated me not to give in when I was sued. There was an aphorism my mother often recited to us as youngsters: "Pride goeth before the fall." Fortunately, I had forgotten that saying when I advised my legal representative to refuse any settlement from the plaintiff's attorney. Otherwise I too, like so many physicians before me and since, would have agreed with the insurance lawyers and avoided the trauma to which I was subjected. But then again, my conscience would not be clear and that would last the rest of my life.

19

Sharon

Sharon's Miraculous Recovery

"You are invited to attend the wedding of our daughter, Sharon."

When we received this wedding invitation my wife asked me, "Who is Sharon Kelley?"

This inquiry was understandable since over the years many doctors, including myself, receive gifts and holiday greetings from grateful patients. However, it's not often you're asked to attend the wedding of a patient whom you haven't seen in over twenty years. This was a young lady whom I first met when she was three days old.

Sharon's forty-two-year-old mother had an uncomplicated full-term pregnancy and normal delivery, but her new-born was having difficulty from the first day.

Dr. Thenebe, her pediatrician, paged me one morning and asked me to meet him in the nursery where he explained the problem.

"This baby is unable to take her formula. She's constantly drooling and having continuous coughing and choking episodes. These symptoms are present even between feedings."

The pediatrician went on to describe similar incidents with other newborns, but their problems resolved in twenty-four to forty-eight hours.

This kind of case was a new experience for me, but I readily agreed to examine Sharon and hoped to find a solution to her difficulty. At this time I didn't realize that many paths would be traveled before this little child would be pronounced as cured.

Under anesthesia, I examined the throat, lungs, and stomach of this tiny infant with our smallest endoscopic instruments. No obstruction or abnormality could be seen that might account for Sharon's failure to swallow without choking.

The next day Dr. Sennett, head of the x-ray department, was consulted and he advised placing some drops of lipiodal into the baby's mouth. Radiologists routinely inject lipiodal into the lungs to discover any abnormality in the bronchial tubes or the lungs themselves. Barium by mouth would cause problems if it followed Sharon's usual pathway of swallowed material going into the lungs.

The dye didn't enter the stomach as normally expected with swallowed substances, but quickly entered the lungs which were clearly and safely outlined. We still had our problem, however, in trying to determine why everything swallowed by Sharon ended up in her lungs.

It was now generally agreed we were faced with an abnormality of the brain center that controls the swallowing reflex. This strange phenomenon sometimes occurs in infants, but usually corrects itself within a few weeks.

Nasal tube feedings were started and this brought her nourishment directly into the stomach. The catheter intake helped to increase her weight, but then Sharon developed another unexpected complication. She was choking many times during the day which was traced to the accumulated salivary secretions. The saliva couldn't be swallowed and drained into her lungs instead. This caused not only choking spells, but also severe attacks of cyanosis which at times were life-threatening.

After two weeks it was necessary to perform a tracheotomy for improvement of her airway and minimize her breathing difficulties. With constant nursing care the tracheotomy opening allowed suctioning whenever the mouth secretions entered the lungs.

Each day we looked forward to Sharon developing a normal swallowing reflex, but our attempts to introduce even a few drops of fluid by mouth caused a severe coughing spell. The feeding tube from the nose into her stomach continued to be her lifeline for full nourishment.

All those entrusted with Sharon's care realized we had reached a point where we weren't making any progress and further consultation was indicated.

During my short period of practice I became acquainted with Dr. Charles Ferguson while attending meetings of the New England ENT Society. This knowledgeable physician was chief of his department at Children's Hospital in Boston. After I explained the predicament of this two-months-old baby he readily agreed to arrange for Sharon's admission and guide her through the steps needed for a full evaluation.

Sharon spent two weeks at the Children's Center before being returned to our care at St. Francis Hospital. The consultants' reports were thorough, but depressing.

One neurologist reported, "She has a serious abnormality of the brain and if she survives it's unlikely that she could maintain an independent existence."

In a final general summary a somewhat hopeless conclusion was given.

"It is our opinion this child cannot survive more than two years and if by chance she does, institutional care will be required."

For several more weeks after readmission to our hospital Sharon failed to show any signs of improvement. It was then decided that a gastrostomy should be done. This opening into the stomach allowed us to remove the nasal tube which was causing irritation of the nose. Even more importantly, substantial feedings could be more readily administered through the use of a gastrostomy tube.

The incision into the abdomen was done by a member of the surgical department. The feeding tube placed into the stomach was much larger than the small nasal catheter. There was a marked improvement in Sharon's general condition, although she did suffer several attacks of heart failure, kidney infections, and bloody vomiting. All these complications were controlled with medications and her progress otherwise continued.

The nurses, who were given the responsibility of her care, never gave up as they continued their daily ministrations. Most outstanding in this attention was Margaret, a middle-aged nurse's aide, who worked the day shift. She became a surrogate mother to Sharon, always being available if one of the shift nurses was unable to be in attendance. Margaret was the one we entrusted with testing her patient's swallowing reflex by offering the baby a few drops of water every couple of days. She shared the doctors' disappointment when she announced the failure of the swallowing efforts.

Sharon celebrated her first birthday at the hospital where she was surrounded by family, nursing personnel, and of course, her doctors. With two other older siblings at home the parents were anxious to know when it might be possible for Sharon to spend some time in her own house. After much instruction the mother felt comfortable in making up the feedings and pumping this life-saving fluid through the gastrostomy tube. Sharon was finally allowed at the age of fifteen months to leave the hospital where she was given a joyous but somewhat tearful send-off.

For the first month Sharon and her mother made the twenty-five-mile trip to my office every week to have the tracheotomy tube changed as well as the dressings around the stomach tube which was left undisturbed.

At the end of that month with no difficulties being apparent the visits were stretched to every two weeks. During each examination I would offer my growing patient several drops of water by mouth. I would also give her a sip of water from a glass in hopes it might stimulate normal swallowing. Her mother was also advised to do the same every few days. All of these attempts ended in failure as the water ended up in her lungs causing severe coughing. I made every effort to appear optimistic with each visit, but without seeing any progress my hopes that this little child would ever be able to swallow normally gradually faded. I found no reports in the medical literature of any youngster developing a normal reflex after this length of time.

At the age of twenty-two months, only one week after her last visit to my office, Sharon's mother called me. Her voice was brimming with excitement.

"I just gave Sharon a few sips of water and she didn't choke or cough. What should I do now?"

"Bring her into the office as soon as you can," I said, feeling the excitement myself. "I'll check her immediately."

Within an hour Mrs. Kelley smilingly ushered Sharon into the office where the entire staff greeted her happily. The other patients in the waiting room were told there would be a slight delay in being seen. The treatment room had been set up for the examination. As Sharon sat in her mother's lap I carefully placed a teaspoonful of water into her mouth. There was no discomfort or coughing or choking as the water disappeared. I then offered her a small cup of water and this too was taken with even greater relish. The smile on her face was equaled only by the satisfaction enjoyed by her mother, her doctor, and the entire staff.

Sharon was hospitalized immediately for more complete evaluations. At the hospital Margaret, the nurse's aide who had spent so much time with this patient, had to be the happiest of all the people who greeted the miracle baby.

A fluid diet was started after admission to the pediatric service and continued for two days.

X-ray examination showed no interference with the swallowing reflexes. The testing barium mixture was seen traveling normally down the esophagus and through the stomach and intestinal tract.

Soft foods were given on the third day and these also were accepted without difficulty. The gastrostomy tube was removed and the stomach opening closed. Then the tracheotomy tube was removed. A week later with the abdominal and neck incisions completely healed, Sharon was discharged from the hospital.

I followed this amazing patient in my office for one month and then discharged her from my care. Since she lived some distance from my office there was no occasion for Sharon to be seen by me. However, I was kept informed of her progress in grade school, high school, and college by her aunt whom I saw regularly for periodic wax removal. The invitation to her wedding after all these years, however, was a complete surprise.

I looked forward to Sharon's wedding and I wasn't disappointed. She was a beautiful, vivacious bride. After the ceremony I felt a warm tingling feeling while meeting all her friends and relatives. They had been aware of the part I had played in Sharon's survival. It was completely overwhelming to hear the words of these young people who thanked me for the help I had given to a dear friend so many years earlier.

In reviewing the developments in Sharon's case, it was obvious she had suffered from an immature swallowing reflex. Case reports indicated if this reflex fails to develop within a few months of birth, the infant usually dies from lack of proper nourishment. The amazing part of the story is how Sharon's reflex center for swallowing finally became normal after two years.

The brain cells work in mysterious ways and the theorists can rationalize as to what had happened. Sharon's family had great faith a miracle might happen and that belief was shared by her doctor.

I often reflect on the number of Sharons we care for, especially in medicine and allied professions. We all seek happiness in this life, but our greatest happiness is obtained in bringing happiness to others. I found my joy in medicine, especially in situations like the miraculous result that occurred with Sharon. However, each and every occupation can be a source of gratification in a person's life, whether it's a professional individual or the common laborer who can bring joy with the simplest of endeavors.

A year after Sharon's wedding her obstetrician, who knew the story of her problems in infancy, informed me she had become pregnant. Naturally she was concerned her child might have the same abnormal reflex she had experienced. Sonograms, which were now available, revealed a perfectly normal fetus and she subsequently gave birth to a healthy baby.

Some years later Sharon told me she was the mother of three healthy children aged two to seven. She expressed her gratitude for my past assistance. I reminded her we all had faith and hopes her recovery would be complete. Despite all the endeavors of the doctors and nurses, we put our trust in the impossible dream called a miracle.

20
Doctors

Doctors Without Compassion

"You must sign these papers before your surgery," the young woman said. "Also it's necessary that payment be made before the operation."

"What are these papers I'm required to sign immediately?" I asked.

"They include permission for the surgery and the reimbursement from Medicare as well as your supplemental insurance carrier. However, payment by you is also required before the surgery is done."

"I can understand the necessity for giving agreement for the surgery, but the immediate signature for insurance reimbursement and payment before the doctor operates seems to be carrying things a bit too far. As a matter of fact I only have a few dollars cash in my pocket."

"Do you have a check?"

"No, I don't have a check."

"Do you have a credit card?"

"Yes, I have a credit card."

"Give me your credit card."

"Tell me, as a physician can't I be trusted to delay all this until the present surgery is completed?"

There was no reply to this request so I sat up on the operating stretcher and signed the required papers. Then I reached into my trousers and extracted my credit card.

This most unusual and discomforting conversation took place in the office of a dermatologist located some seventy-five miles from where I lived. The referral had been initiated a week earlier by a dermatologist near my home whom I saw because of a suspicious skin lesion on the side of my nose.

This skin specialist was recommended by a physician friend. He agreed the nasal growth appeared malignant and took a biopsy. He also advised consultation with a surgeon trained in the Mohs technique for skin cancers and I agreed to follow his suggestion. Several days later the skin doctor called to confirm that the nasal tissue was malignant and the appointment was made to be seen by his recommended surgeon.

The visit to the consultant dermatologist developed into a series of unexpected and somewhat traumatic events. A keratotic, thickened skin lesion on my right cheek had been present for several months and the consultant advised removal of this, also. It wouldn't require the Mohs technique and I agreed to its removal by the usual type of excision.

My primary concern was the growth on my nose which was the reason for consultation with the dermatologist. While the surgeon examined this nasal lesion we reviewed the background of Frederich Mohs, the originator of this unusual approach some fifty years earlier. Having read extensively about this type of microscopic excision I was able to relate why, as a physician, this type of surgery appealed to me.

The modern development of magnification allowed the surgeon to remove a malignancy without wide excision of tissue. This is especially important when surgery is performed on the nose and near the eye. The Mohs surgeon then brings the removed specimen into the adjacent laboratory and examines the edges under the microscope to determine if cancer cells are present. When malignancy is found close to the edge of the resected tissue then additional surgery is required immediately.

After the surgeon examined the area on my nose using a magnifying loupe, I was satisfied the Mohs technique should be done and this surgeon was qualified to perform the operation. However, the nasal surgery which requires several hours or more couldn't be booked for another month. The surgeon suggested the removal of the cheek lesion could be done at this present visit since it was only a half hour procedure and didn't require the microscopic technique.

It was after the injection of the local anesthesia for the cheek lesion that I was literally attacked by the secretary in the presence of the surgeon. My protests about immediate payment were ignored and I decided to make no further comment until the thickened-skin surgery was completed.

I felt sufficient rapport had been established with the surgeon and all questions about the microscopic technique were answered satisfactorily. Before leaving the office I was given an appointment for the nasal cancer surgery one month later.

On returning home I expressed my dismay to the referring physician for the manner in which payment was demanded prior to surgery. The doctor insisted the consultant dermatologist was well trained and had an excellent reputation. My concern, as I emphasized to him, was the manner in which payment was demanded.

The secretary's request for payment had ended by surrendering my credit card. At no time was any suggestion made to allow paying the balance of the bill after the insurance coverage was received. Medicare and my secondary supplemental medical carrier would guarantee the surgeon adequate compensation, but this physician wanted immediate payment for the cancer surgery. No consideration was given to me, an eighty-year-old patient, and also a physician.

The lesion on my nose had been present for several months, but only in recent weeks had it appeared like something more than a simple benign growth. I decided, as with any cancer, that it was important for definitive surgery to be done without any further delay.

One month later I arrived at the consultant dermatologist's office thirty minutes ahead of schedule and was told surgery would be delayed. When my appointed time came and passed I finally asked the secretary why there was such a prolonged waiting period for my surgery.

"The surgeon has a patient with a melanoma and as a doctor yourself you know that must be taken care of immediately."

Melanoma can be a problem for the surgeon and the patient, but after the date for my cancer surgery had been put off for a month, the unexpected delay at this time was understandably upsetting. Melanomas don't develop overnight, but I said nothing further.

Although the postponed starting time for surgery increased my anxiety for the cancer operation, the atmosphere in the operating suite made me more uncomfortable. There was a definite chill in the air and I realized my protests to the Hartford dermatologist had probably been channeled back to the surgeon and the assistant.

The technician draped me for the surgery and prepared the table of operating instruments. There wasn't any communication while the surgeon became gowned and checked the equipment.

My attempt at a pleasant "good morning" was not acknowledged and the surgery was begun. The failure of the surgeon to acknowledge my presence or offer even a weak apology for the delay was unexpected. Whenever my patients were subjected to a long delay in the office, which occurred occasionally, an explanation and regrets were given. Despite the unresponsive cool atmosphere, I decided to continue my efforts at breaking down the wall that had been established.

My next attempt at interrupting this disturbing silence occurred during the operation when I asked, "How is everything going?"

There was no response from the surgeon again which increased my mental discomfort. On my first visit during the removal of the thickened-skin growth we had a pleasant interchange. At that time it was a discussion about the technique used for the removal of the cancer on my nose. Now that this procedure was being done I was anxious to be kept abreast of how things were going.

Several years earlier I had undergone prostate and major ear surgeries under local anesthesia. It was reassuring as a physician to be kept informed of what was going on. The surgeons involved were kind enough to answer my questions. Despite my concern about the eventual diagnosis and outcome of the tissue removed in these operations I was completely relaxed by their responses while the procedures were being done.

Some patients, especially those involved in medical care, such as nurses and physicians, often are more comfortable when they can reach out to their doctors with questions during the operation. Nonmedical individuals are more likely to request that they be put to sleep and learn the results after surgery. This is understandable.

I repeated my question, "How is the operation going?" several more times during the operation with no response from the surgeon.

In the meantime the surgeon and the technician carried on a somewhat inane conversation about places they had recently visited. This total silence in response to my inquiries while being subjected to nonsensical bits of conversational trivia increased my annoyance.

After the surgery of several hours duration was completed the surgeon did a complete disappearing act which mystified me. Although this was an office procedure, the operation was not the removal of a simple cyst but a significant malignant tumor. I expected the surgeon to give me a few minutes of time after the operation and explain what had taken place.

After waiting for several minutes, I approached the secretary.

"I am concerned about the surgery and the tissue report," I said, "and I'd like to speak to the doctor."

"The doctor is busy with another patient," she said without looking up.

"When can I see the doctor?"

"The doctor has a long operation and won't be available for several hours."

I had arrived at his office at 9:30 AM and between the delay in starting the operation and the intervals necessary to examine the removed tissue, it was now well after 1 PM.

My wife, a registered nurse, had accompanied me to the dermatologist's office realizing the surgery would take several hours. The postoperative dressing would also involve a bandage covering one eye so I wouldn't be able to drive. Her Irish temper finally got the best of her and she insisted she wanted to discuss the operation with the doctor. However, the same infuriating response given to me a short time before was now given to her.

"The doctor is busy with another patient."

For any patient to be treated in this manner is demeaning, but to subject an elderly physician and his wife, a nurse, to this type of rude behavior really defies description.

On returning home, I dialed the surgeon's office and asked to speak to the doctor. I was informed that the sugeon wasn't available. I left my number and asked to be called. After several days of no response I made several subsequent calls after office hours in the hopes the surgeon might be available. The answering service had the same answer each time I called.

"The doctor will call you back if it's an emergency or you should make an appointment to be seen."

I never received a call back.

I returned to the office a week later for suture removal. Another delay of more than an hour occurred beyond my appointed time. I was first placed in a treatment room for this procedure and without the sutures being removed I was then asked to return to the waiting room.

"Why can't this be done now so we can get it over with?"

"We have an emergency and your case isn't urgent."

Half an hour later I was returned to the treatment room for the suture removal, but another problem developed. The technician, without the surgeon's assistance, spent many minutes clumsily trying to remove the sutures. The surgeon was finally called from another room and took one look and announced that the lower half of the wound had failed to close.

"It will be necessary to resuture the incision but absorbable sutures will be used this time which will not require removal."

There was no other conversation.

As the surgeon silently began to prepare the necessary needles and sutures, I looked up and said, "Aren't you going to anesthetize the area?"

"It won't hurt," was the response. "It's just a pinch."

As the needle was inserted into my skin, I couldn't restrain my feeling of discomfort.

"Damn it all," I blurted out, "that needle hurts. Put in some local anesthesia."

The surgeon came back with the same answer.

"It doesn't hurt. It's just a pinch."

The suture needle was inserted six times on each side of the long incision before I was informed that the repair was finished. The tears that flowed from my eyes were partly from anger and partly from pain.

I never subjected any patient of mine to such barbaric treatment and I had never experienced this kind of pain at the hands of any physician or dentist during my entire lifetime.

After this final humiliating encounter I refused to accept an appointment for further evaluation. I didn't wish to be subjected to any further indignity from such a completely insensitive physician.

Five months after payment of the services had been billed to my credit card I decided to contact the dermatologist's medical association in the southern part of the state. Complete credit had not yet been received by me from Medicare or my major medical coverage, but I had fulfilled my total financial obligation by payment to Master Card.

In my correspondence to the medical association's evaluation committee I detailed the actions that had occurred during my visits to this insensitive physician. At the same time I also gave an itemized report of the amount received by me from Medicare up to that point.

It was my hope the letter to the medical association would result in a reprimanding note to the physician. I wasn't interested in bringing any legal action since that wasn't my reason or intent.

The responses received by me from the medical association were completely defensive without any acknowledgement of improper conduct by the surgeon. In response to my explanation of the fees charged and payments made by Medicare up to that time, the committee had what appeared to be a pat answer.

"The charges by the surgeon are reasonable. The allowed payment by Medicare results in an out-of-pocket expense to you of $487, not the $1055 you claimed."

Anyone with Medicare experience knows the amount allowed isn't what is paid. The committee was accusing me of cheating. That certainly was an indication as to what the rest of their responses would be.

Prior to the first surgery I was appalled by this doctor's callous treatment of a patient, especially an eighty-year-old physician. To me it was a total lack of common decency. Practically every physician of my acquaintance treated older citizens with kindness and respect.

The fact I was a retired physician was known to the surgeon, but no special reduction of the fee was asked even though it was of gigantic proportions. There wasn't any attempt by me to ask that the charge be reduced because of my status as a physician. What did annoy me was the demand that I should "pay up front" and I considered this demeaning to me as a member of the medical profession.

In replying to my letter of complaint the medical association's review committee gave their interpretation of what had transpired.

"The surgeon didn't realize you were a physician. The doctor's secretary explained the billing policies at the first appointment. You never asked for assignment and you never mentioned any financial difficulties."

The surgeon's statement claiming to be unaware that I was a physician was a deliberate falsehood. When writing to the medical association I had explained that I had discussed my background as an otolaryngologist with the surgeon and this had taken place during our first meeting. The medical association, by accepting the surgeon's claim of not knowing I was a physician, obviously implied I was lying. The statement about financial difficulties was totally uncalled for since it indicated in essence that I was claiming to be a pauper.

Their evaluation committee also ignored my concern and annoyance regarding the demand for payment of a very large fee before the surgery was performed. I stated this exorbitant charge was outside the range of normal fees charged by other doctors and was an unfair request for any senior retiree. There was no mention of this by the committee.

In my letter I expressed discontent at the unusual delay for the second and third office visits. This was a relatively minor inconvenience which I accepted, but I stated an attempt should be made to avoid such a waiting period or at least minimized for elderly patients. The county committee went to great lengths in reminding me that as a physician I should be aware of delayed appointments. What the committee didn't acknowledge was the surgeon's failure to make even a weak apology for my delayed appointments.

After receiving the response from the committee I had the mistaken idea a review of my comments might cause some change in their thinking. My second letter of protest questioning the results of their decision was answered four months later. I assumed this review committee was either very busy with a heavy caseload of complaints or simply didn't care.

The committee's reply was brief and definitely disturbing to me as a physician.

"Your correspondence was reviewed and our committee believes their conclusions were correct and were rendered in an unbiased manner. The committee considers the case closed."

I realized that any reprimand of the offending physician, even a slap on the wrist, wouldn't be considered by the medical association's evaluation committee. My only reason for challenging the surgeon was to question what I considered impropriety in demanding payment prior to surgery, failure to communicate with the patient at the end of surgery, and more importantly, complete lack of compassion. There wasn't any intent and I never sought any action to deprive this physician of the right to practice surgery. There was no desire on my part to bring suit or any other legal force against this doctor.

My main concern was that the actions imposed on me were unconscionable, not simply because I was a physician, but because I was a human being and a senior retired individual.

Since the billings assessed on me appeared definitely out of line, I reviewed the charges the surgeon submitted to Medicare. It was clearly evident that an overcharge was made. This prompted my decision to seek further investigation. I realized the medical association's evaluation committee would reject any suggestion the billings were out of line. They had already closed the case.

I contacted the Program Integrity Section of Medicare and I was told to outline what errors might have been made in the surgeon's billing to Medicare. After several telephone conversations I was requested to give a detailed description of the surgical procedures that had been performed.

As a physician with knowledge of this microscopic surgery there wasn't any difficulty in explaining what had been done and where obvious false charges had been made. I presented an outline of the steps involved in the surgery.

"In the Mohs technique the borders of the removed tissue are examined for any possible tumor cells. If cancer is found then further resection is done and the edges of this second removal are examined for malignant cells. The second resection by the surgeon was found to be negative and the surgeon closed the wound. However, in my review of the billing I noted the surgeon charged for a third resection which was not done."

After receiving my letter there were once again calls from the Medicare Integrity Section before final action was determined and a decision made as to the amount of overcharge.

"Our Medicare medical director has reviewed the medical records and the overcharges are hereby noted. The total amount of the billings by your surgeon amounted to $3,135.87. The amount allowed to be collected from you is $1,200.78. A refund of $1,935.09 has been requested from your doctor. Thank you for bringing this matter to our attention."

Within a few days a check was received from the dermatological surgeon and finally this unfortunate episode in my medical life came to an end.

In reviewing the events that transpired, including the responses of the physician's medical association, I was deeply disturbed by all these developments. The final financial adjustment received by me took place fifteen months after the original charges had been made on my credit card.

Knowledge of the steps involved in the Mohs technique allowed me to identify exactly what had been done and what had been billed to Medicare. Individuals who weren't acquainted with that type of surgery would have had little likelihood of questioning the billing statement. The possibility of such overcharging is overwhelming.

After reviewing my experience with the surgeon's medical association I could readily appreciate how a complaint from a deserving patient may sometimes face difficulties.

Having served on county committees myself, I can assure any aggrieved individual that proper consideration is usually given to all who seek help. At times a committee may be pressured into actions by a favored group that wants to protect its own turf. The defense of the medical association, accepting that doctor's word as the truth and mine as false, was extremely upsetting.

During my years of practice and since retirement it has become necessary to seek the attention of a number of physicians for a variety of ailments. On occasion some of these problems appeared life-threatening. Depending on the symptoms, physicians were consulted in Boston and Connecticut, and after retirement it was occasionally necessary to consult doctors in Florida.

On one occasion in Florida, a skin lesion developed near my eyelid. I was referred to a surgeon trained in the Mohs technique. The treatment was carried out effectively with acceptance of Medicare coverage and the payment by my supplemental medical insurance. The Florida physicians extended the same warm professional approach I had always received from doctors whose advice and treatment I requested.

My fifty years as an otolaryngologist are filled with happy memories. As with any successful practitioner the steady stream of patients was generated by referrals from others who had received treatment from me. The care I extended to those who came to my office was the same kind of attention and concern I expected to find when there was need for relief of my own symptoms. The doctors I consulted were personal friends or physicians recognized for their professional competence. I never failed to express my gratitude by a note of appreciation.

It came as a shock to have the bitter experience of undergoing surgery at the hands of an uncaring physician. What was more appalling was the response of the dermatologist's medical care evaluation committee. My intent was merely to change a physician somehow who had no sense of compassion. This obviously failed.

The committee's attempts to condemn me were totally unjustified. More disturbing was their willingness to accept the surgeon's conduct as perfectly legitimate. Their replies to my correspondence left me with the feeling they embraced such actions by the physician. That is a sad commentary on the deliberation of any medical association whose primary responsibility is to examine complaints in an unbiased manner.

I directed the attention of the dermatologist's medical association to my appointments and election as an officer to local, state, and national societies of my specialty. Such accomplishments, of which I was justifiably proud, were completely ignored as apparently without substance in their opinion.

Since retirement I'm appalled by the low fees paid by Medicare for the medical charges submitted by my personal physicians. These doctors spent a considerable amount of time with me, as they do with all their patients, and yet their payments are comparable to unskilled labor. The excessive charges by some physicians and medical equipment suppliers are now being examined more closely. In many cases they have been found to be fraudulent. Undoubtedly moneys channeled into the hands of dishonest individuals and groups diminishes the availability of funds for the honest practitioner.

For many years prior to the establishment of Medicare and Medicaid, it was the responsibility of physicians to render free service to those unable to pay for private medical care. This included patients seen on the ward service of the private hospitals as well as staffing the local municipal medical facilities. Our commitment to these institutions for many months each year was done without expectation of compensation. This was accepted as the norm for our dedication to the profession we hold in such high regard.

Perhaps the new social approach of assuring medical care for everyone has changed the perspective of a few physicians as to their true objectives. With my three children involved in medically allied services, including one son actively practicing internal medicine, I am keenly aware of the problems facing the medical profession.

Albert Schweitzer, the world-renowned physician, dedicated his life to the care of the medically-deprived inhabitants of Africa many years ago. He made a statement that should be the guidepost for all physicians.

"We should become better human beings, more humane than we are."

The dermatological surgeon's lack of respect and dignity accorded to me as an eighty-year-old patient was humiliating and disappointing. The review of the Medical Evaluation Committee compounded the hurt that I experienced. Certainly if this type of attitude was adopted by all review committees the medical profession would face justifiable accusations from all interested community groups.

Compassion is the one quality all patients seek when they visit their doctor. The members of the medical profession continue to be revered and placed on a higher pinnacle than any other group in our society. This attitude can only be maintained if there is a sincere and unbiased evaluation of a patient's complaints. A review committee has a moral responsibility to the aggrieved patient as well as to the accused physician.

Doctors, Medicare, and Fraud

Universal health care for Americans was first suggested by Theodore Roosevelt in 1912. It was also proposed by Franklin Delano Roosevelt in 1935 and signed into law by Lyndon Johnson in 1965.

The first full year of Medicare in 1967 cost $3.3 billion. By 1990 this had grown to $107 billion. With the number of individuals living to age 65 and older increasing rapidly, the cost of Medicare has expanded dramatically. The prophets of doom anticipate that not only Medicare, but also Social Security will go bust.

Each day the pages of the daily newspapers bring reports of fraud being perpetrated by those entrusted with the medical care of our citizens. The biggest headlines are usually reserved for the physicians who have been caught and found guilty of falsifying charges. Unfortunately these losses are minimal compared to the illegitimate billions being taken by the huge HMOs that have wrested control of medical care from the physicians in this country. These super conglomerates have taken over management of massive numbers of patients and doctors frequently by devious means. When their profits fail to satisfy the executives and stockholders, they cut down the compensation to the doctors. And it's odd how their computers seem to "break down" allowing them to delay payments to physicians.

An amazing number of technical groups have been born with the advent of Medicare. Many individuals have been induced to sign up for equipment that is useless or unneeded. All of this seems to escape the eyes of investigators until the untold loss of millions has been uncovered. During times of financial crisis experienced by the conglomerates the salaries of their major officers continue to soar into the millions.

The consumer who has been promised the "pie in the sky" is the ultimate victim since the treatments or diagnostic evaluations recommended by their physicians are often limited or even refused. Untrained employees are deciding essential therapies aren't warranted and the powerless patient is forced to continue with his suffering. As more and more of such cases become publicized there will be a demand for the honest doctor to have greater discretion in treating the very ill patient. Don't expect any change in the near future since those in charge of these huge groups are not about to give up their "territorial rights" nor their inflated incomes.

Overcoming Roadblocks in Medicine

"Be not the first by whom the new are tried nor yet the last to lay the old aside."

Alexander Pope wrote these words over 250 years ago, but for many centuries before his statement and for years ever since, physicians have sought to break through the resistance set up by the traditionalists who favored the "status quo" approach to treatment instead of accepting new ideas.

In the mid 1800s the experience of Pasteur was almost doomed to failure as he fought against the odds while developing the method of partial sterilization of liquids now called Pasteurization, and the development of the rabies vaccine. His scientific colleagues resented his success and were slow in accepting his results.

Edward Jenner was severely criticized and condemned by the Royal Society of London when he requested publication of his paper on smallpox vaccination in the late 18th century. He was forced to publish the article at his own expense. The treatment was then adopted in France, Russia, and America. Acceptance by his British colleagues didn't occur until recognition by those outside his own country.

During my years of practice I was a follower and not a leader. By being a conformist I was able to avoid the pitfalls that occur when you go off the beaten path and adopt some totally unacceptable kind of therapy.

If something new in the way of treatment in surgery or medicine was brought to my attention, however, I didn't close my eyes and ears to the alternative approaches. If my medical readings or attendance at scientific meetings indicated there was merit in a different attack on a specific disease I investigated the problem more deeply. When the new approach offered promise of helping my patients I would seek out the seminars and instruction courses for further knowledge. After gaining reassurance from these sources, I then followed the new direction in the care of my patients.

In the specialty of ear, nose, and throat I found the welcome mat was always out when visiting the pioneers of the newest procedures either in their offices or the operating rooms. These steps often convinced me to adopt or reject the procedure being advocated.

Allergy and the Shot Doctors

"The RAST is now being utilized by otolaryngologists, chiropractors, osteopaths, and others."

This report from the medical association was instantly challenged by a number of otolaryngologists. The committee's report was distributed to the members of the association at the behest of several general allergists, but without the review or approval of any otolaryngologists. The grouping of chiropractors 'and others' with otolaryngologists was a blatant attempt at smearing those ENT physicians who used this test. It was also an endeavor to convince insurance carriers that the test wasn't valid.

"Did you read the latest reports from the medical association?"

This call to me came from a fellow otolaryngologist.

"No," I said. "I've been away for the past week and haven't checked my mail."

"Well, you should read it over, since the family allergists are trying to prevent you and other otolaryngologists from doing any RAST testing."

Dripping noses and nasal congestion have always been a common problem with patients seeking advice and treatment from the otolaryngologist. Nasal sprays and packings as well as the newer decongestants gave relief to many of the victims.

In some cases skin testing was performed by family doctors practicing allergy with desensitization injections given at regular intervals of one to four weeks and continued for many years. The patients were often told that failure to maintain the schedule could result in the development of asthma.

During one summer season when the pollen count was extremely high I decided the resistant cases might be improved by skin testing and injections of the offending allergen. A number of otolaryngologists had used the low dosage approach successfully and were restricting their practice to ear, nose, and throat allergy.

After several years of successfully treating patients with the minimal dosage method a new concept for allergic diagnosis was introduced by Japanese and Swedish researchers.

This radioimmunoassay test (R.A.S.T.) offered a simple solution to the patient's allergy problems without subjecting the individual to multiple skin pricks. It was especially adaptable for children who resisted the repeated needle injections. The test also appealed to adults who preferred not to spend several hours in the physician's office having skin tests done followed by a waiting period for the response to be read.

Not only the ENT physicians, with many years of practice devoted to allergy, but many other physicians decided to look into this new advance for diagnosing and treating allergies.

This became a problem for the family allergist who made his decision for treatment on the basis of his past training and experience. That method involved as many as several hundred skin injections on the patient's arms and back. A charge was made for each needle prick which raised the cost to many hundreds of dollars.

If the RAST was used as a screening test the cost would result in considerable savings to the patient. This was true not only for the testing, but also by avoiding the unnecessary treatments resulting from false positives of the multiple skin tests.

The RAST required only a single skin prick for a blood sample. The technician then placed this blood specimen in a special apparatus purchased for testing the patient's blood. The test took twenty-fours to develop and it offered an alternative method of diagnosing allergies.

After attending a number of scientific sessions where the RAST was thoroughly explained and demonstrated, I decided to include this advanced technology in my allergy practice. I also continued to use the otolaryngologist's standard method of skin testing for diagnosis.

There had been no complaints from the general medical allergists about the ENT method of diagnosis and treatment. When one of the family allergists decided to retest his patients with the RAST rather than skin testing, however, his charges for RAST were severely inflated.

Based on the use and charges for the RAST by that one general allergist, the other members of his group were correct in condemning the RAST procedure as expensive. The local insurance companies were advised by these unhappy allergists that medical coverage shouldn't include any payment for the test which they claimed was ineffective.

In a scathing report, the ethics committee of the county medical association followed up this misrepresentation of the facts with more attacks on the RAST. They bluntly stated this was a controversial test performed by unqualified physicians. This report was sent to all the members of the association from a committee headed by a retired former general allergist.

The accusations were especially vicious in stating ENT specialists weren't qualified to treat allergy patients. This was extremely annoying to the otolaryngologists who never voiced any complaint about the general allergists treating sinusitis patients. After all, the practice of medicine allows the patients to choose their doctors. The attempt by the family allergists to blacken the character of the otolaryngologists was too much for the ENT specialists, even those who didn't include allergy testing in their practice.

At the insistence of the American Otolaryngic Allergy Society, of which I was a member, a meeting was arranged with the Aetna Insurance Company's medical director. Following this formal gathering it was agreed by the Aetna Medical Department that the RAST was an acceptable and reimbursable procedure. A limiting allowance of $100 for the test was decided upon as a fair but restrictive compensation. In many cases this would eliminate the need for many hundreds of skin tests which the family allergists performed. Other insurance carriers followed suit. There weren't any further complaints from the general allergists.

One of the precepts I learned as a youngster was "when you stop beating your head against the wall it feels good." I was happy that my efforts helped to bring changes in what had become an autocratic approach to medical treatment by one group of self-centered physicians. It was disturbing to spend many hours appearing before committees who had already made up their minds as to what they considered right.

Shortly after that ordeal was successfully concluded a young ophthalmologist was threatened with suspension from the medical association by refusing to lower his fee for detached retinal repair. This highly-trained eye specialist had opposition from a few of his fellow ophthalmologists and an insurance provider. The complaining doctors were not professionally equipped to perform this highly technical procedure. The accused eye physician's expertise was gained by additional years of training in this delicate operative approach. He confidently brought his case before the state medical society where he was completely vindicated.

Allergies are now more widely controlled with oral medications obviating the need for injection treatments. The RAST, as with tests for thyroid and other blood sample procedures, has gained wider acceptance where allergy evaluation is indicated. Its simplicity and accuracy has reduced the costly method of approach that had been relatively unchanged for over 75 years.

There is no question that skin testing has a place in diagnosing allergic disorders, but as in other forms of alternative treatment the choice should be a decision by the physician and patient. It shouldn't be determined by doctors with tunnel vision who refuse to broaden their views of what is best for the patient.

The chest physicians haven't always supported allergy shots in the past. They believe they have the ability to control asthma and related pulmonary problems much more efficiently with advanced medications. This is again in keeping with the advances in medical knowledge and the changes possible with alternative treatments.

In commenting on the controversy created by the family allergists, Dr. Harold Schuknecht, a world-renowned otologist whom I mentioned before, offered a profound statement.

"There is a feeling by some physicians that their specialty is protected turf that cannot be invaded by interlopers. The changes in medical practice by outside agencies will certainly have an impact on the acceptance of some treatments that may have been shunned in the past."

Patients are now much more knowledgeable and cost-conscious. They receive a vast amount of information from medical sources through the media and the Internet. The patient must beware of the charlatans in our midst. This is especially true for the victims with diseases that defy the efforts of our best medical experts.

Bulbar Poliomyelitis, A Fight to Save Patients' Lives

"I am sorry to bother you, Dr. Curran, but the medical doctor asked that you do a tracheotomy on a patient in the iron lung."

The emergency call came from the Contagion Unit at the City Hospital in Hartford on a very hot July 4th afternoon in 1955. When I arrived at the hospital the bulbar polio patient was gasping for air despite the assistance of the pulmonary machine known as the Drinker Respirator named after its inventor.

As I prepared to do the surgery the nurse supplied a brief history.

"Mrs. Mahoney was admitted from Torrington three days ago. She was seen by the polio physician shortly after coming into the unit."

"How was her breathing at that time?" I asked.

"She was having a lot of difficulty and I asked Dr. James if I should call you about doing a tracheotomy first. He became very angry and told me he would make that decision so I said nothing more. Her breathing has been getting worse even though we've been suctioning her throat as much as possible."

When I gazed at the thirty-three-year-old mother of three children there was no question this was another case of doing too little too late. The nurse attending Mrs. Mahoney was suctioning the mouth secretions, but the patient's color and diminished chest movements indicated it was a losing battle. The catheter couldn't be inserted deeply enough to be of any use. It was a repetition of the cases on whom I had been asked to do a tracheotomy during this epidemic bulbar polio season.

The incision in the neck for a tracheotomy is a relatively simple procedure, but when performed on a patient in the iron lung it does present a few problems. The patient cannot be removed from the respirator on which she is totally dependent. Even a few minutes out of the iron lung could bring death.

When Mrs. Mahoney was encased in this huge apparatus only her head and neck were exposed. The chest and abdomen moved up and down to keep the lungs active as the respirator did its work.

The epidemic of bulbar polio affected the breathing center of the brain and produced a staggering mortality despite the use of the respirator. The paralyzed chest muscles couldn't be sufficiently stimulated by the respirator to overcome the secretions accumulating in the lungs. The nurses vainly attempted to clear the airway by suctioning the mucus from the patient's throat. Their suction catheters couldn't reach down into the trachea and into the lungs. Gradually the weakened chest muscles deteriorated to the point where the respirator couldn't force the fluid from the lungs. The patients literally drowned in their own secretions.

I did the tracheotomy on Mrs. Mahoney using a local anesthetic since endotracheal anesthesia hadn't been developed in the early 1950s. With the cuff of the respirator moving up and down against my hands, I made the incision over the midline of the neck. The trachea was exposed after separating and tying off the overlying blood vessels. A bleeding artery in cases like this could be fatal.

As soon as I made the incision into the trachea there was a burst of air and secretions immediately filled the opening. The assisting nurse quickly suctioned them off. The insertion of the tracheotomy tube finalized the procedure. The nurse pushed her suction catheter through the airway tube deep into the lower lungs and pulled back massive amounts of thick, tenacious mucus. The patient's lips which had a bluish hue up to this point now showed a pink coloration.

Mrs. Mahoney, who couldn't speak because of the tracheotomy, moved her lips saying "thank you." Her eyes told me what she felt.

Although she was feeling comfortable because of her easier breathing, I knew she was probably thinking of her three young children at home, hoping she could return to them once more. I wanted to share her anticipation of happiness, but having gone through the frustration of delayed tracheotomies before, there was considerable doubt in my mind. In the past whenever the tracheotomy was performed there was a temporary improvement, but the ravages of this terrible disease would drain the patient's breathing reserve and the patient inevitably expired.

For two days after surgery the nurses continued to suction out huge amounts of mucus. This gave them hope their efforts would be successful. The patient's chest movements, however, became weaker as the muscle reserve lost its power. On the third day while making rounds I approached Mrs. Mahoney's bedside. I noticed the apprehension of the nurses as the polio physician placed his stethoscope on the patient's chest. He then turned and lifted his head.

"I hear no heart beats," he said. "Mrs. Mahoney has expired."

Most of my cases requiring tracheotomy involved children with croup. The results were almost always dramatically successful. Bulbar polio patients seen by me were young adults, most often female, and were almost terminal when tracheotomy was requested. Despite the instant improvement following surgery the ravages of the disease had been allowed to progress too far and very few patients survived.

While leaving the polio unit later that morning I again saw the physician who had been supervising the care of the patient who had expired. I decided this was the opportune time to express my feelings.

"Dr. James, I know you are just as disappointed as I am by Mrs. Mahoney's death. You must realize if we are going to save lives it's essential that I see these patients earlier for tracheotomy to give these patients a better chance to overcome their disease."

The response was about as I had expected. He addressed me in his most authoritative voice, letting me know he was in complete charge.

"Young man, I have been in practice for many many years and have devoted much time and effort in helping individuals who have been attacked by this disease. You have been taking care of nose and throat problems for only a few short years and have practically no experience in treating polio patients. What right have you to tell me when I should call for your consultation?"

The response of Dr. James upset me for a few seconds, but I decided to come right back at him.

"Your objectives and mine are the same, the survival of the patient. I admit that your knowledge and experience is vastly greater than mine, but I'm being asked to attend patients with breathing difficulties who are close to death. All I'm requesting from you is an opportunity to see and evaluate these patients as soon as they are admitted and not when there is little chance of survival."

Dr. James gave me a withering glance, said nothing more and then abruptly turned and walked away. I realized he wasn't going to change his ways no matter what I said.

Several weeks earlier, while attending a meeting in Chicago, I was captivated by an address given by Dr. Thomas Galloway. This tall, white-haired, distinguished doctor had become so disturbed by the death rate from bulbar polio he decided to devote all his efforts to finding a solution for this devastating disease.

"Early tracheotomy is the only solution for bulbar poliomyelitis if we are to reduce the mortality rate of 90%. After many months of animal research our group has advocated and performed tracheotomy as soon as the patient has been admitted. We have reduced the mortality rate to 40%."

I approached Dr. Galloway after his presentation and poured out my laments.

"I'm seeing too many individuals who live only a few days after tracheotomy. Most of these patients are placed in the Drinker Respirator shortly after admission to the hospital. I'm never asked to see them until their condition has almost become moribund. What can I do to convince the doctors tracheotomy should be done early?"

"Some doctors are hard to convince," Dr. Galloway said. "But they have to be reasonable and willing to share the successful experience of others. You have a stake in the patient's survival and the polio physicians must recognize that your views are important. Their patients are experiencing a 90% mortality as we did before performing early tracheotomy. Meet with them and show them what our group has accomplished."

Infused with his enthusiasm I returned home with Dr. Galloway's message of hope. I decided to take a more forceful attitude in promoting early tracheotomy. The death of Mrs. Mahoney and my confrontation with Dr. James stirred me into immediate action.

My first step was to review the charts of all the patients who had been seen by me for tracheotomy. In each case I had strongly advised that these desperately ill polio victims should have been seen earlier, preferably on the day of their admission. All my efforts in these cases had been futile since my notes failed to persuade any of the attending physicians to consider early surgery.

The warm summer months of 1955 had caused an unusual number of patients to be afflicted with the bulbar disease. All the stricken victims were admitted with marked dyspnea (difficulty breathing) and were placed in the iron lung shortly after admission or sometimes several days later. I was called only after the patients got much worse.

At this time there wasn't any specific medication available to treat the polio virus. As in the past the nurses' efforts to clear the airway were continually frustrated by their inability to do anything except remove mucus from the throat. In the cases that eventually underwent tracheotomy the nurses were encouraged by their success in removing the deep secretions and temporarily making the patients more comfortable. Their notes written on the patients' chart suggesting earlier tracheotomy were ignored by the attending physicians.

When reviewing the records of the patients I had seen for tracheotomy I was also able to gather information on all those admitted with polio. Some of those patients had died but were not referred for possible tracheotomy. Most of my anger was triggered by the realization that ten of the twelve patients seen by me had died. They had failed to survive despite my surgical efforts. I decided to bite the bullet. I would demand an overall change in the treatment protocol for all patients admitted with the diagnosis of polio. I knew this would cause turmoil in the thought processes of those physicians who refused to accept any modification of their time-honored, but fatal concepts of treatment.

I called upon an orthopedic friend, Dr. O'Connell, for advice.

"Maurice, as a member of the City Hospital staff I'm often asked to see polio patients who have breathing problems. However, the victims of this disease have little chance of recovery by the time the request comes to me for tracheotomy. The attending physicians are giving me the brush-off when I ask them to call me sooner to perform the surgery."

"As an orthopedist," Dr. O'Connell said, "I have nothing to do with the patients who have breathing problems, Tim. Those physicians in charge are knowledgeable individuals and have years of experience. I suggest you direct a letter to the chairman asking for an opportunity to present your views. I'll contact him personally, and you should attend our next monthly meeting. Don't expect too much from these doctors since a lot of them have a 'know it all' attitude."

My letter to the chairman of the polio committee was acknowledged and I was asked to attend their monthly meeting two weeks later. It was now necessary to review the charts of the patients admitted to the contagion unit with the specific diagnosis of bulbar polio. Since this type of polio was almost epidemic during the six months of my summer service

I was the only ENT physician who was asked to see these patients.

On the night of the meeting the only familiar person I saw was Dr. O'Connell. I felt like a duck out of water. The other members present were from other area hospitals so I was a complete stranger to them. While looking around at the twelve members surrounding me, I had the uncomfortable feeling they were the jury (which they were) and I was the one who was being judged. To a great degree this was true.

During the dinner, which was served prior to the formal meeting, I had little in the way of conversation with anyone except Dr. O'Connell. From the quizzical looks directed at me I wondered whether I was just wasting my time.

It came as a relief when the dishes were cleared from the table and the chairman, Dr. Smith, gave a few introductory remarks. After receiving acceptance of my request to appear before the committee I had sent a brief resume of my training and military service. The chairman made no mention of my background and therefore I was an unknown to the majority of those present.

Reading from notes and also speaking extemporaneously, I detailed the progression of the patient's symptoms in each of the twelve cases I had reviewed. The nurses' bedside notes were especially revealing since they documented what I had been stressing to these same physicians whenever we discussed their patients.

The reports written by the nurses were quoted verbatim.

"The thick secretions have been suctioned from the mouth. The patient's breathing continues to be labored since the mucus deep in the lungs can't be reached. The tracheotomy procedure would at least allow us to clear the obstruction to the lower breathing passages."

Knowing the nurses' notes would be more effective than anything said by me, I emphasized what they had written.

"These are dedicated nurses," I continued, "who have been given a great responsibility and they are constantly frustrated in their attempts to make the patient comfortable and save that person's life."

I described how ten of the twelve patients died within two or three days, the surgery having prolonged their lives only another twenty-four to thirty-six hours.

"The patient's life was hanging by a thread when the request was submitted for emergency tracheotomy. I knew and the nurses knew that only by early tracheotomy could they reach the depths of the lungs with their catheters necessary to save the patient. That was the only way to help prevent the victims of this disease from drowning in their own secretions. I want all of you to realize this is something the nurses and I truly believe that tracheotomy is not only the best but also the only solution to this catastrophic fatal disease."

To bolster my position I held up the book on bulbar polio written by Dr. Galloway.

"This is the story of how Dr. Galloway decreased a 90% mortality rate to 40%. After I spoke with him I was sure we could get the same results. We are all devastated with the terrible loss of lives caused by this modern-day plague, but I assure you we can and will do something about it."

After finishing my presentation I asked if there were any questions. The first person with his hand up was Dr. James whom I had confronted several weeks earlier.

"Don't you think, Dr. Curran, that perhaps your tracheotomy hastened the death or even caused the deaths of those patients?"

There were approving nods from several physicians in the audience, but I decided this wasn't the time for me to become angry and lose my temper.

"The victims of this dread disease were already at death's door when I first saw them. That's the reason why I'm here today. If I had been called sooner and had become a part of the decision-making team we could provide a better service to the patient. Being asked to perform a tracheotomy when the patient is at death's door isn't fair to the patient or to me."

This response stimulated further questions from my audience, but as the session ended I sensed a feeling of defeat. The physicians present were polite, but displayed no enthusiasm for accepting a somewhat innovative approach. I thanked them for their attention and departed from the meeting room.

The following day I met Dr. O'Connell at the hospital. He told me there was considerable discussion among the committee members after I left. Many recognized a change in the treatment protocol was necessary. The only question by some members was whether the recommendations of a young physician with little knowledge of bulbar polio should be accepted or other avenues be sought.

About a week later I was called to see a thirty-year-old male bulbar-polio patient with severe respiratory difficulties. The attending physician asked for my evaluation before the young man was placed in the iron lung. I examined the patient and quickly performed the necessary tracheotomy. He was then encased in the respirator to help his paralyzed breathing muscles.

The nurses were ecstatic as their suctioning efforts were rewarded immediately by easily clearing the lungs of the secretions. The catheter introduced through the tracheotomy tube gave instantaneous improvement. Instead of a deterioration of the patient's breathing in the next few days this polio victim gradually improved. He eventually made a complete recovery and was discharged to home care about six weeks later.

My service ended some two months later. During that time I saw four more cases requiring tracheotomy. I examined all of these patients shortly after admission and before they were placed in the iron lung. Only one of these patients failed to survive although he lived for a few weeks before succumbing to the disease. The other patients required the assistance of the respirator for several months, but early tracheotomy helped to prevent the deadly effects of pneumonia. They recovered sufficiently to leave the hospital and continue their medical care at home.

The polio vaccine developed by Dr. Jonas Salk in 1953 was safely used on several million volunteers in 1954. The testing program initiated at the University of Michigan in 1955 gave impetus to the almost universal program of vaccination in this country and throughout the world. The incidence of polio cases dropped dramatically and became almost non-existent after 1956.

My services for the care of bulbar polio patients no longer were necessary. I must admit to an early disenchantment when I first proposed tracheotomy as a positive solution for this terrible disease. The eventual acceptance by some physicians willing to follow this approach taught me the importance of fighting for a principle. You can sometimes overcome the negative thinking of others, but you must also learn to accept rejection and not give up. You can only change contrary opinions by continuing the battle when you know you are right.

EPILOGUE

When Faith Overcomes Adversity

When my brother John developed paralysis of the leg at the age of three, as I described at the beginning of this book, there was no noticeable change in his condition for many months despite medical attention and massage therapy. Following visits to the "Church of Miracles" it would have been difficult to convince my mother that anything but divine intervention brought about John's complete recovery.

Coming from humble beginnings and overcoming the pitfalls encountered by low-income families is not unique for many who have reached a degree of success. There are few who can truthfully say they are completely self-made. Along the way to achieving the goal they had set for themselves there was someone who reached down and helped to pull them up the ladder. The one constant instilled in our young family was the faith of a mother who believed the Lord was always there when help was needed.

There were many who gave members of our family guidance and opportunities in those early years of struggle. John took his job as the surrogate father very seriously. He was a continuing stimulus in encouraging us to keep looking ahead. He had to face his own struggle to gain an education and reach his goal of becoming an attorney, but there was always someone there who stretched out a hand of support. His own aspirations didn't deter him from lending help to the other siblings until they were assured of success in their endeavors.

Maintaining my position as a drugstore clerk couldn't have been accomplished without the kindness and affection of Fred Archer, the owner of the pharmacy. This employment from the sixth grade through the second year of medical school guaranteed my financial salvation and provided the stimulus to seek a future in medicine. That included the period of the Great Depression with joblessness that affected millions. Many of the people were forced to seek welfare assistance. Our family was able to survive and found no need for further recourse to the public support that had provided us with basic sustenance for two years after my father's death.

When I think of helpful angels my thoughts always go back to Dr.

Roswell Ham who assured my entrance into Boston University Medical School by his letter of recommendation. He really was heaven-sent as I recall the diminished chances of reaching my goal as a doctor if Dr. Ham hadn't strongly endorsed my application for admission.

As one goes through life the ravages of disease are faced by all of us. The fact we escape so often is a tribute to the great advances in medicine. There are some cases where it appears unlikely that the victim will survive and yet he does survive. The recovery is often believed by the patient and family to be a miracle. The doctor frequently has no answer for the unusual phenomenon that may occur.

It came as a total shock to me when densities were noted in one of my lungs after routine chest x-rays at the time of an annual physical. My anxiety increased with each succeeding week as more shadows were seen on follow-up x-rays. The radiologists, chest specialists, and other consultants were equally baffled as to the exact diagnosis.

By the time the eight week arrived and new nodules were being seen, there appeared to be no hope of survival. The complete lack of any symptoms, despite the widespread dissemination of shadows in both lungs, was puzzling to me and my doctors.

When the chest films showed gradual clearing and finally complete disappearance of the shadows in the ninth and tenth weeks all the physicians involved in my case had no answer as to the cause or the cure. My family and all our intimate friends who knew of the undiagnosed threat to my life constantly reminded me of their spiritual support. They were just as certain as I that their prayers were a strong factor in my recovery.

In more recent years such an event might be ascribed to something in the immune system. This theme has become popular with some caretakers who have followed patients with malignant diseases that disappear spontaneously despite apparent failure of treatment to stem the progress of a cancer.

Christian Scientists are strong in their belief that faith heals. They refuse to seek medical help for their diseases in many instances.

Dr. Herbert Benson, founder of The Mind-Body Institute at Beth-Israel Hospital in Boston made a profound statement after several years of observation where patients were noted to make unusual recoveries from their illnesses.

"I am not a religious person," he wrote, "but I came to my belief not from religion, but science that caused my feet to drag."

Benson advocates the use of such techniques as the Relaxation Response which he promoted in his teachings along with standard medical practices.

As I pointed out in describing all the tests and examinations during my ordeal, I saw no reason to take a course of antibiotics since I had no fever or cough and my blood counts were completely normal. Any such treatment would have been given the credit for the cure, but I agree with my family and friends that the Lord made his presence known. There doesn't seem to be any other explanation for the spontaneous disappearance of the threatening lung shadows.

When my little patient, Sharon, failed to develop a normal swallowing reflex after several weeks, the outlook was grim. After one year without improvement it was difficult to maintain a glimmer of hope she might ever eat and drink normally. During that period of time she had been examined thoroughly at one of the world's leading pediatric medical centers and these consultants found no reason for optimism. The development of the reflex at two years of age defies scientific explanation.

Christian Scientists rely solely on prayer to guide them on self-healing journeys.

Perhaps Dr. Benson expresses it best when he said, "I cannot envision a world without penicillin or surgery. It would be just as onerous to say you don't need drugs and surgery as to say they're the only approach you need."

Addendum
Some Unforgettable People

Woody and Dr. Whalen

Chester Woodford was his given name, but there were few who ever knew him except by the salutation "Woody." He had served in the armed forces during World War I and that included many months in overseas duty. He never spoke of his war experiences, but he was always entertaining with his social conversation. Woody had a flaring mustache and a hair-styling that gave him a debonair appearance.

His travels in Europe included a romance with a lady he referred to as the "Countess" whom he married. She was the mother of his only child, Knud. Woody became a good friend because he had a pleasing personality and belonged to the "AA" (always available).

Within the first few months of my practice he invited Mary and me to join him for dinner and reminded us to "bring the baby." These invitations came often and knowing Woody, I'm sure they were spontaneous without ever consulting his affectionate and ever-dutiful wife. Our son Timothy was only a few months old, but Woody and Ann, his second wife, made us feel like longtime friends.

Whenever I had scheduled a long or involved surgical procedure, Woody was always available to lend a helping hand. In my early years of practice, physicians didn't belong to groups and only rarely did doctors have other associates working with them as partners.

It was especially helpful to ask Woody to cover any of my emergencies when I attended a meeting out of town or spent a few days on vacation with the family.

I never knew him to lose his temper or say an unkind word about anyone. He didn't have a large ENT practice which was probably the way he preferred it to be. He had an unusually gifted pair of hands that made him an excellent asset whenever he assisted on a surgical procedure.

His lifelong friend was Dr. Whalen. Their close association dated back to their first years of practice. Although Woody admitted to many romances and two marriages, his friendship with Dr. Whalen (Eddie) survived the passage of time. Dr. Whalen was a member of all the prestigious medical societies locally and nationally. His erudite manner and depth of knowledge were recognized not only in the ENT specialty groups, but also in the state medical society where he was elected president.

Dr. Whalen encouraged me to learn the new procedures that were rapidly developing in our specialty following WWII. With his stimulation the path to the newest treatments became a must rather than let's wait and see. The demands of maintaining a rapidly increasing active practice and a growing family required a lot of sacrifice to spend several days and sometimes weeks at seminars where the leaders of ENT taught us the latest developments.

Dr. Whalen remained a bachelor throughout his lifetime, prompting me once to inquire, "Why haven't you ever married?"

"Nobody ever asked me," he said.

As a family we frequently invited Dr. Whalen to join us for birthday events or impromptu affairs with friends. He always accepted these offers and never failed to make the evening much more enjoyable and instructive by his comments.

Since it was this inspiring physician who helped to guide me into becoming an otolaryngologist, I've always felt since he was a bachelor, that he took a fatherly interest in me and my family. This was occasionally evident when he would counsel me in words that I should utter or directions I might take during my years of practice.

Sunday mornings I frequently took my preschool son, Timothy, on my rounds to the hospital. On one occasion I found it necessary to reprimand Timothy and emphasized this by tapping him on the backside.

Dr. Whalen didn't approve.

"That's not the way to take care of the situation," he said.

He was absolutely correct. I learned from a bachelor that talking to the child is a better approach no matter how mild the physical punishment might be.

Woody and Dr. Whalen were two doctors whose encouragement and support helped to make my life as a physician more enjoyable and rewarding. They remained steadfast friends and when each passed away in turn, I was at their bedside grieving over them.

Two Devoted Nurses

The nuns ran St. Francis Hospital from the time of its inception until my retirement and beyond. They were a completely dedicated group who helped to strengthen the position of the hospital in the community and surrounding areas.

The operating room, however, had two stalwart nurses who were not nuns but gave as much service and affection as any member of a religious order could give. Nora Walsh and Mary Smyth ran surgery, although there was a nun who theoretically was in charge. These two ladies supervised the scheduling, squeezed in the emergency cases, and let the doctors know they, Nora and Smitty, were running the show.

Occasionally it became necessary to penalize a surgeon who was periodically late for his elective cases. The placement of his surgical procedure infuriated some of the offending doctors. Although the nun in charge made the decision it became the responsibility of Smitty and Nora to confront the delinquent doctor.

These two firm and efficient nurses not only kept the schedule going smoothly, they also were the official greeters of each patient who arrived in the operating room. They introduced themselves, reassuring each and every one of these individuals they had nothing to worry about. No matter how serious the planned operation might be, they left the patient with the feeling everything was going to be smooth and uncomplicated.

Over the years these truly inspiring nurses had built up such a tremendous rapport with so many patients that arrivals in the operating room for the first time looked forward to meeting them. Word of mouth had alerted one and all that Smitty or Nora would be there to say hello. They had no need for a public relations department. The patients, some with repeat visits, were just as anxious to have a friendly greeting from them as they were to see their surgeons.

A Nun's Story

"Wouldn't it be nice to have a cold glass of beer today, Sister?"

"It would be, but herself does not approve of it."

Sister Patricia worked in the kitchen of our hospital during my internship and she was still continuing her duties upon my return to Hartford to begin my ENT practice. This good nun had left Ireland some fifty years before I first met her. She still had an Irish brogue "thick enough to cut with a knife" as the expression was used in Boston.

As internes we would occasionally be delayed in the operating room or detained elsewhere in the hospital because of some emergency. We'd seek out Sister Patricia who was always in the kitchen.

"Sister, what do you have for a hungry man?"

Her beckoning finger would lead us to the walk-in refrigerator.

"Follow me," she'd say. "I can see you have been working very hard today. Tell me what you would like and I will fix it up right away."

Whether it was a choice of steak, chops, or chicken, we were given our selection along with any of the available vegetables.

"How would you like me to cook it?" she'd inquire.

In a short while the prepared meal was brought to the table and then she would hesitate for a few minutes until I had sampled the food.

"Does it taste all right for you?"

Once she was assured everything was perfect she would depart to her other duties.

This delightful nun literally dragged herself along since she was hampered by a long-standing arthritis and a curvature of the spine that didn't allow her to stand or sit up straight. Yet she never failed to greet everyone with a smile whenever you met her morning, noon, or night.

It was during my first year of practice, while passing by the kitchen area and heading for the doctors' dining room, I noticed Sister Patricia resting in the area reserved for the nuns. It was an unusually hot day in the middle of a very hot summer and yet Sister was carrying on her duties with the same benevolent smile that never left her face. There wasn't any air-conditioning in the kitchen area nor in the rest of the hospital in those days.

I exchanged greetings with Sister Patricia and commented on the hot weather and was just about to continue on my way when I thought that perhaps a cooling refreshment was in order. When Sister made the comment about "herself not approving beer as a refreshment," I said nothing further and went on to the dining room for lunch. "Herself" was the Mother Superior whom I recalled vividly during my interne days. She was an excellent administrator but quite rigid in her rules. This lack of flexibility was resented by many of the practicing physicians and especially by the internes in our group. She had complete control and didn't hesitate to exercise that power to the limit.

After finishing lunch I started to think about Sister Patricia and how dedicated she was without ever asking or receiving little or nothing in the way of material blessings. Before I went to the office I decided to do something that might bring an unexpected bit of joy to this devoted nun.

I hurried over to a nearby liquor store and purchased a six-pack of cold beer and asked them to put it in a bag so no one would suspect it contained beer.

In a few moments the liquor store owner returned with the bag of beer.

"How about this Lord and Taylor bag?" he said. "My wife had a new pair of shoes in it."

Carrying the shopping bag of beer, I made my way to the secluded alcove in the basement of the hospital. Sister Patricia was seated by herself having a cup of tea.

"Sister, I have some cold beer I think you might like. Enjoy it in good health as we say in Ireland."

The broad smile on her beaming face told me I had done the right thing as she grasped my hand and said, " Thank you, Doctor, thank you very much."

As I left she raised her arms in a blessing for me, again expressing her gratitude for my little gesture.

It was several days later while passing through the kitchen area I caught the eye of Sister Patricia seated in the nun's enclosure. She gave me a big wave and then motioned with her finger for me to come in. As she sat at the table with the usual teacup in front of her, I stood at a respectful distance.

"Have you had a chance to try the beer, Sister?" I asked.

With a twinkle in her eye and a broad smile on her face, she pointed to the teacup.

"Yes," she said, smacking her lips, "and I am having some this very moment."

Years ago we often heard the story of the nun who would have her martini in a teacup. In those days the nuns were dressed in their clerical habits and it was a cause for scandal if they were seen drinking in public. Sister Patricia was the first nun I ever knew who successfully accomplished that little subterfuge.

During that very hot summer I was able to replenish Sister's supply of beer at regular intervals. This grateful nun always expressed her appreciation and never failed to say, "I offer a prayer for you every day, Doctor."

Near the end of the summer I learned Sister Patricia had been transferred to the infirmary located at the Mother House several miles away. Her increasing arthritic problems no longer allowed her to carry on her kitchen duties.

It was several months later that a notice appeared in the hospital bulletin reporting the death of this wonderful, dedicated nun. This was not unexpected since Sister Patricia was well into her 80s. She undoubtedly had multiple ailments in addition to her extreme arthritic condition.

When I recalled how grateful she had been, I had one lingering regret. I just wished I had made a trip to the infirmary and presented her with one final ice-cold six-pack of beer. Sister Patricia would have enjoyed such a gesture, I am sure.

A Japanese Friend

Ruri Wada became a part of my medical life shortly after she arrived in the United States. Her husband, Don, was given a one-year assignment by his Japanese company to work at Monsanto Chemical located in the suburbs of Hartford, Connecticut.

Ruri, who had very little knowledge of English, decided she needed to keep herself occupied in some endeavor that would be beneficial, but not require too much oral communication. She offered her services to St. Francis Hospital as a volunteer and was assigned to the linen room where she folded material that was being readied for use in the operating suite.

Her work table was located just inside the wide door that faced the corridor connecting the operating pavilion with the doctors' dressing rooms. While folding her linens she could observe the doctors and other personnel walking by. If their eyes turned towards her she greeted them with a smile and a gentle wave of her hand.

After several such pleasant greetings, I discovered stopping by to say hello was rewarded with a more expansive smile and obvious joy. These almost daily encounters became more gratifying as her command of English increased and she was no longer limited to the words 'hello and OK.' When St. Patrick's day arrived I visited the hospital gift shop and purchased a card and green carnation which she proudly pinned to her uniform.

Just before Ruri and her husband departed for their return to Japan, our son Tim finished his tour of duty as a combat marine in Vietnam. A welcome-home party was attended by friends, neighbors, and various individuals from the operating room where Tim had worked several summers as an OR technician. We also invited Ruri and her husband. Ruri now could move easily among the other guests with no difficulty in communication.

Her departure home didn't diminish the friendly ties that had been established. Christmas card greetings were followed by yearly letters as we kept each other informed of family events such as the births of her two daughters and her son. My correspondence with Ruri kept her up to date about the doctors and nurses whom she knew at the hospital as well as describing the marriage of my son Tim and later his brother John.

Eventually her daughters, Nagisa and Akane, were given an opportunity to study in California and New York. Later her son, Nanahiro, attended college in New York.

The children's educational pursuits became an incentive for Ruri and her husband Don Wada to visit the United States again, including several trips to the Hartford area. These trips eventually allowed us to meet all the children who were just as gracious as their parents. The Wada's host family, Hugh and Sally Meinweiser, with whom they lived during their one-year stay in Hartford, also renewed their friendship that has continued after this delightful Japanese couple went back to their homeland some twenty-five years earlier.

Becoming a close friend of Ruri and then her family was an experience that was joyfully shared by my wife and children. It helped us to realize that reaching out to others brings mutual respect and trust that unites people in a common bond. This is a heritage that exists throughout the world, but is often ruptured by the political self-seekers looking for personal glory.

When Old Surgeons Fail to Make the Cut

"All surgeons who have reached the age of sixty-five will be required to submit to a physical and mental examination if they wish to maintain their operating privileges."

This bombshell was dropped by the chairman at a monthly meeting of the surgical department. There hadn't been any prior discussion or consultation with the department heads of the surgical sub-specialties such as my own. The unexpected declaration apparently came about as a result of a recent article in the College of Surgeons Bulletin recommending this requirement be instituted for all members of the surgical staffs over the age of sixty-five.

Dr. Mannix hadn't even finished his statement when several of the subspecialists began to voice their discontent. In most cases those who were approaching or past the age of sixty-five became the spearhead of opposition to the age requirement. One of the older general surgeons with a very active practice stood up.

"This is a crazy idea and I demand that it be dropped immediately."

The younger surgeons struggling to build up their practice remained silent, but it was obvious they could see some of the older men walking the plank. The chairman realized he had opened a can of worms, but he was determined to see the whole thing through. After a little calm had been established, the meeting continued in an orderly manner.

It was recognized the hospital had a retirement policy already in effect for its employees. Why shouldn't the surgeons also be willing to accept the inevitability of retirement and submit to an annual evaluation?

This sounds reasonable on the surface, but doctors have always prided themselves on being individualists. To be told they were going to be carefully scrutinized for their fitness to continue as surgeons seemed to infringe on their freedom and rights.

Before going on to discuss the age cut-off, I suggested all staff members should be included. Certainly the internists, pediatricians, chest physicians, cardiologists, and other non-surgical physicians had the same responsibility to patients as the surgeons and they should all be included if the evaluation was to become official. This opened another discussion which became heated as one more question was posed.

"Why pick an arbitrary age of sixty-five? Perhaps the age cut-off should be fifty and that will include our chairman."

This caused much sputtering by the surgical chief as well as those in the fifty-year age bracket.

Subsequently, this latter suggestion was withdrawn since the statements were made partly in jest. The decision regarding the cut-off age was, for the time being, wisely put aside.

The next question was how the evaluation would begin. It was agreed the first step would be the physical examination. At this point I stood up again and recalled my experience with routine chest x-rays.

"Several years ago during a routine physical examination my chest x-rays showed densities that didn't clear for almost three months. Would such a finding now place my surgical privileges in jeopardy?"

The difficulty in determining standards for the physical exam paled into insignificance when we started to tackle the mental evaluation. Partly in a humorous vein, one doctor posed a question.

"Would a surgeon lose his right to operate if he walked into the operating room with his fly unzipped or gravy on his vest?"

As one get older, the doctor, just like other people, may develop a few such peculiarities. Do these quirks interfere with his ability to perform the work satisfactorily? There was also an uneasy feeling grapevine gossip might contribute to the grading of one's emotional stability.

Also discussed were the criteria that would be used in assessing the performance of the surgeon in the OR. There would have to be some objective tests that must be employed to measure the individual's ability. The mortality rate of patients undergoing surgery as well as the number of complications and the length of operating time are all simple and useful determinations, but such gauges were already in effect and applied to all surgeons.

How about asking the operating room supervisors to be the first line of offense in judging the surgeon's skill and ability? Are nurses really appropriate judges of the surgeon's skill and ability? It was finally determined that only physicians should judge their colleagues.

We still had to be concerned as to the method of dealing with the doctor who failed to meet the standards that might be set up. Should the physician have his privileges curtailed or should he be forced off the staff altogether? Some of the committee members felt uncomfortable about informing a colleague he was no longer acceptable. They didn't wish to visualize themselves as being hatchet men looking to cut off the head of a long-respected associate.

Before the meeting broke up, the committee did agree that any mandatory evaluation of the older surgeons would include all the physicians on the staff and not be restricted to the surgical service.

As I walked out of that meeting the handwriting on the wall became more evident. Being a doctor who had just reached the age of sixty, I could feel a hand on my shoulder. I knew it was Father Time telling me that soon I might have to face up to a retirement I might not want.

Nothing ever developed from this meeting except in a very general way. The climate was in evidence that the older surgeon, at least, was going to be under closer scrutiny. It became the primary responsibility of the department heads to see that each and every operator was closely watched, if not supervised, especially if complications occurred.

The importance of this was realized four years earlier in our department. One of the surgeons had a mild stroke that caused some weakness in his hands. He was anxious to continue surgery which could have placed the patient in some jeopardy. Unfortunately, some of his doctor friends encouraged him to resume his surgical activity. As the department chief my refusal to permit him to operate created resentment and some unpleasantness. I stuck to my guns, but for a short period of time I lost the friendship and the referrals from several of my colleagues.

Several months after the surgical meeting I wrote an article that was accepted for publication in Medical Economics, the national medical magazine. It was entitled, "Old Surgeons Never Die and That's The Problem."

Like old soldiers, the old surgeon should also realize that although he too may want to continue to fight the battle, he must just quietly fade away.